W. L. Macke

Health and Disease

SE**V**ERUS
Verlag

Mackenzie, William Leslie: Health and Disease
Hamburg, SEVERUS Verlag 2011.
Nachdruck der Originalausgabe von 1911.

ISBN: 978-3-86347-120-0
Druck: SEVERUS Verlag, Hamburg 2011

Der SEVERUS Verlag ist ein Imprint der Diplomica Verlag GmbH.

Bibliografische Information der Deutschen Nationalbibliothek:
Die Deutsche Nationalbibliothek verzeichnet diese Publikation in der
Deutschen Nationalbibliografie; detaillierte bibliografische Daten sind
im Internet über http://dnb.d-nb.de abrufbar.

SE**V**ERUS
Verlag

CONTENTS

CHAP.		PAGE
I	WHAT IS HEALTH?	7
II	THE CAUSES OF DEATH—THEIR NAMING AND CLASSIFICATION	23
III	DEATH-RATES AND THEIR INTERPRETATION	41
IV	FEVER, INFECTIOUS DISEASE, AND EPIDEMICS	52
V	STUDY OF A TOXIC INFECTION AND ITS ANTITOXIN	79
VI	HOW ANTITOXINS ARE PRODUCED AND PREPARED	91
VII	IMMUNITY—NATURAL AND ACQUIRED .	100
VIII	A DISCUSSION OF THE TUBERCULAR DIATHESIS	114
IX	THE ADMINISTRATIVE ASPECTS OF TUBERCULOSIS	134
X	THE INTERNATIONAL INFECTIONS—PLAGUE, CHOLERA, AND YELLOW FEVER . .	155
XI	OTHER PREVENTABLE DISEASES . .	170
XII	THE HYGIENICS OF A STAPLE FOOD—MILK	180
XIII	THE HOUSE AS IMMEDIATE FAMILY ENVIRONMENT OR HOME	197
XIV	DISEASE AND DESTITUTION . . .	214
XV	INSURANCE METHODS OF PREVENTING SICKNESS	220
XVI	THE EVOLUTION OF THE HEALTH MOVEMENT	231
	NOTE ON BOOKS	253

HEALTH AND DISEASE

CHAPTER I

WHAT IS HEALTH ?

" AND what a strong, healthy man he looked ! " This was the comment at the funeral of a burly farmer. He was of middle age ; ruddy in countenance ; muscular ; of large bone, deep chest, irrepressible activity. His laugh was strong and clear. His eye was active. He knew no fatigue. He took more than his share in business, in social life, in public affairs. From the cradle, he had enjoyed good nurture. In his youth, he had been an all-round athlete. As he grew older, he turned his energies to the more complex matters of life. Every one said of him,— " Here is a strong, healthy man." Yet, under fifty, he suddenly took pneumonia and in three or four days was dead.

" What a thin, pale creature he looks ! " This was the common remark about a dis-

tinguished physician. Like the farmer, he
had come of good stock. He had been well
nurtured in infancy. He had enjoyed all
the advantages of physical and general
education. But he had always been more or
less high strung and " delicate." He had
been persevering and studious at College ;
he became an accomplished man ; he had an
eye for details ; he had skill in speculation.
Early in his day, he set himself to analyse
the conditions of long life. He concluded
that the climax of health was a healthy brain.
The condition of maintaining it he found to
be regular habits of food, sleep, and exercise.
He established, by a study of his own nature,
certain normals of life. These, once determined, he kept to rigidly, seeing always
through the day to the day after. He decided
that to maintain elasticity of brain was a
greater total gain than to go under to the
impulses of the hour. In a word, he fulfilled,
as nearly as the conditions of climate, education, and duty permitted, the aims of the
" simple life." He lived at low pressure. He
achieved a great reputation. He died at the
age of ninety-four. In this country, such an
age is accounted " advanced."

These two are extremes. But let us look
round on the society of every day. Here is
a beautiful child of ten. From earliest

observation she was called clever. She was always in advance of the children of her age. She came rapidly to the front at school. She was alert, keen, energetic. Her blue eyes were bright ; her complexion pure " pink and white " ; her eyelashes were long ; her form was slim and thin. You could see the blue veins in her temples. She was in fact a perfect specimen of the " fairy " type. But, in an outbreak of diphtheria at school, she caught the disease and died within a week. After death her body was found saturated with tuberculosis.

Or again, take note of this lithe, handsome man, the incarnation of activity, ready-witted, fit for great work in any line of life. He is full of splendid schemes. He is perhaps somewhat boastful, outraging his friends by the extravagance of his ideas, embarrassing his enemies by the cleverness of his intrigues ; talking, inventing, travelling, gathering experience from every civilisation. But he carries within him a remnant of a terrible infection. He may die suddenly, or pass through a long vegetative life in an asylum. He may live for years ; but, with his present record, no insurance company would accept his life.

Or turn once more to contemplate this stalwart, self-possessed, learned man, who,

able and moderately persevering, has come
healthily forward through the forties into the
fifties. He has not stinted himself of the
good things of life ; but he has never been
seriously ill and never had to miss either a
day's work or a day's enjoyment. See him
again a year later. What is it that has
dethroned the expression of his countenance,
the mastery in his action, the purpose behind
all his days ? A small swelling appeared at
the side of his tongue. At first he thought
nothing of it ; then, being a doctor, he began
to have uneasy suspicions, but put away a
certain obsession ; at last he took courage to
submit himself to a surgeon. The diagnosis
was — cancer. Within a day, the surgeon
excised the tumour. For somewhat more
than a year, there was no recurrence of the
growth. But soon a slight swelling began to
appear in the glands of the neck. In less
than a year more, he died of exhaustion.

And so, through illimitable variations,
man after man, sooner or later, comes to the
gates of death. Health ? Disease ? What
are these ? In all the cases described health
seemed to be the name for the personal condition ; yet in every case disease was already
in possession. The powerful farmer died of
strenuous living, going down like a felled
ox after a night's chill exposure, because

the pneumococcus, the infective agent of pneumonia, suddenly found the conditions that enabled it to move from its harmless colony in the mouth into the wider ranges of the bodily system. The old physician, by living at low pressure, watching with care the organs of absorption and excretion, under-eating rather than over-eating, never over stimulating, lived on nearly to a hundred, and died of " old age." If Metchnikoff, the wizard of the Pasteur Institute of Paris, be right, old age is a genuine disease. Even in this careful physician, it had probably begun before middle age ; it crept stealthily on until function after function was impaired ; it ended by starving out of their energies all the nutritive director cells of the brain. " Advancing old age " takes, in the world of Metchnikoff's ideas, a perfectly definite, con-crete meaning. It means a progressive dis-ease of the arteries, and it necessarily ends in death. The pretty young child any doctor would at once recognise as a case of tuber-culosis—a subtle parasitic infection, which is not incompatible with the most brilliant mental achievements. Indeed, sometimes it has been maintained that the toxins of tuberculosis are, at certain stages of life, a potent stimulant of latent nerve energies, and may, within limits, be an ultimate advantage to the individual and the race. This is speculation ; yet so complex are the problems of health that no speculation may be lightly set aside. Then the lithe, panther-like man, whose energies seemed inexhaustible, had contracted syphilis in early days. It had been imperfectly cured ; it had affected his arteries ; it had affected his nerves ; it had paved the way for general paralysis.

These are cases of apparent health. How shall we test the reality ?

Let it be said at once that, in the absolute sense, there is no health. What we so name is entirely relative to the conditions of life. If a man remained perfectly " healthy," he would live for ever. But no man lives for ever. It follows that no man lives a complete life of perfect health. The idea of absolute health, therefore, may be cast aside as an illusion, a mere working concept, an ideal that is unrelated to reality. It comes of our invincible tendency to project our hopes on the screen of the future. The tendency, being a necessary illusion, will continue for all time to do its work in each generation. It is the note of youth, when the claim to health is strongest ; it is the note of middle age, when the fear of lost health begins ; it is the note of mature age, when the memories of youth begin once more to predominate. None the less science has no place for an ideal of absolute health. All that science, which is the sum of experience, permits us to entertain, is a normal balance of functions relative to a place in the world.

If you would know how this normal is determined, how real it is in the business of life, look over carefully the health-schedule of a life insurance company. There, when a man asks to be insured, he will find himself regarded from a hundred standpoints. The object of the insurance is to make easier, by co-operation, a money provision for his old age. As the world must go on, men die one after another, not all at once. Out of this simple fact the insurance companies, working by elaborate systems of probability, provide immense benefits for the man's old age without any fear of a bad debt. But, to do so, they must take only " selected lives." It is in the selection of the life that the insurer finds in how many relations he stands to the society that makes an insurance on his life possible. His whole object is " money on easy terms." The insurance company's whole object is " long life to the applicant."

Let us glance at some of the questions

asked. He must declare his age, his occupation, his residence, often his race and
nationality. He must go back over his
personal life and declare all diseases, great
and small, that he has suffered from. He
must detail his habits of food, of drink, of
work, of relaxation, of exercise, of travel.
He must, in a word, sketch, in terms of
common life, all the conditions that affect,
negatively or positively, his probable length
of days. But the record does not end there.
He is closely questioned about his father,
his mother, his brothers, his sisters, his
relatives on the father's side, his relatives
on the mother's side, and he must declare
all the diseases they were known to suffer
from ; whether they were healthy in living ;
if dead, what the causes of death were ;
what the length of illness was ; what their
circumstances in life were ; their nurture,
their education, their localities ; what their
exposures to danger and disease have been,
and as many other details as a " full family
history " should contain. In a word, he
must give data for an estimate of his
" heredity." Further, he must satisfy the
examiner as to his future. He must indicate where he is to live,—in a temperate
climate or a tropical climate, in a healthy
country or a country full of disease. If he

is to go abroad, he must give data for estimating the future risk of exposure to malaria, tuberculosis, plague, cholera, yellow fever, and the mass of other fatal tropical diseases. If he stays at home, he must tell whether his occupation shall be indoor or outdoor, healthy or unhealthy.

But, in all this, the examiner is merely accumulating data for an estimate of probability. He accepts, for what they are worth, the statements of the applicant. He will now put them to the test. To test his food habits, he examines the teeth, the tongue, the stomach, the liver, the bowels. He goes systematically over every physiological system of the body,—the skin, the muscular system, the alimentary system, the circulatory system, the respiratory system, the nervous system. He examines the heart and blood-vessels directly. He tests and records the heart sounds ; he tests and records the rate of the pulse, its regularity, its pressure ; he tests by special apparatus the general blood-pressure. He examines the lungs minutely, back and front, above and below. He tests their resonance, the incoming and outgoing of the breath, the presence or absence of pleurisy, of bronchitis, or pneumonia, or tuberculosis, or any other condition affecting respiration.

He cross-examines the applicant on all his past ailments. He overhauls the nervous system, — motion, sensation, co-ordination. He examines the joints, too, and satisfies himself of the healthiness of every bone or practically every bone in the skeleton. And so he passes over every organ of the body, testing each for any condition that might tend to shorten life. Even this does not end the examination. The examiner tests the secretion of the kidneys ; for some form of kidney disease is not incompatible with temporary appearances of health.

When the examiner marshals his data, he is able, from the wide range of experience now available in organised medicine, to estimate the chances of long life. The insurance companies, basing their scrutiny on a still wider experience of recorded life and death, fix a margin of safety, and so arrange their benefits that there shall be no loss on the total. That, on the whole, they succeed, is obvious from the history of insurance. That, on the whole, they give satisfaction to the insurers, is obvious from the steady extension of insurance methods. But it is on the infinitely careful scientific scrutiny made possible by modern medicine that the immense superstructures of these financial institutions have been reared. To

them, health has, therefore, a concrete
significance. They are " men of business."
They mean to make health " pay."

But the applicant for insurance believes
himself to be without physiological flaw.
He may be undeceived ; but he may be
confirmed. In either case, it is health he
seeks to prove. But he is not the best subject for analysis. True, no man is entirely
normal ; but health can be best understood
from its contrast. Let us consider a case
of disease.

What does the physician ask when he is
called in ? If he is systematic and the patient
is a stranger, he finds out substantially the
same details as the examiner for insurance.
They are all relevant to almost any illness ;
but they are not all of equal importance in
a given illness. Many of them may, therefore, be taken for granted or ascertained at
leisure. The problem of the moment is not
to accumulate data for an estimate of probability ; it is to analyse a problem with a
view to immediate action. The physician,
therefore, is punctilious as to the length of
the illness, the day it began, when it became
severe, when it reached, in the patient's
feelings, the climax that urged him to summon
the doctor. He notes, silently, the posture,

the expression, the complexion, the state of excitement or collapse, and the multitude of other fine shades that only experience enables a man to recognise. These signs, minute though they be, are of immense value. The face, as it appears in enteric fever, has one expression ; as it appears in typhus fever, it has another ; as it appears in plague, it has yet another. Each of them has a significance for the skilled observer. To an old physician the face tells a hundred tales. He has read them a thousand times. He knows every shade of meaning from " the soft play of life " to the terror of the last agony. A gallery of the faces of disease would represent every shade of tragic expression.

When he is satisfied of his dates, the physician comes closer to the facts. He asks about pain, about exposure to infection, about the regularity of habits, about food, about work, about exercise. Then he proceeds to experiment. He feels and counts the pulse ; he watches and counts the respirations ; he takes the temperature. By these he is guided to particular examinations of lungs, of heart, of kidney, of nervous system, of digestive organs. Perhaps he makes no diagnosis of a definite disease ; but, from his scrutiny, he can tell whether disease is present or not.

On what presuppositions does he proceed ? His questions have each a definite purpose. Each presupposes a normal condition, and he is seeking to ascertain if there is anything abnormal. When he counts the pulse, he assumes that, in the adult, the pulse-beats number about seventy to the minute. But he knows that the pulse, even in normal health, varies rapidly. It may be affected by nervousness, by the sudden increase of the patient's attention, by a passing fear, by the posture, by a recent meal, and by many other circumstances. All these he allows for ; but from the simple contact of the finger, he can learn the rate, the rhythm, the volume of blood passing through the artery, the force of the impulse that drives it, the length of each wave, and the wave variations. He can ascertain the blood-pressure, which is of primary physiological importance. He can know directly whether the arteries are diseased or not. He can judge provisionally whether the heart is normal ; whether the temperature is raised ; whether poisons are affecting the system, and an endless variety of other points. But all presuppose a normal pulse.

It is the same in the temperature experiment. If the temperature of the body exceeds 98·4° Fahrenheit (37° Centigrade),

he looks for some special reason. Fever
begins when the temperature exceeds 99°
Fahrenheit. The temperature of the body
varies between well-ascertained limits,—normally, in the morning it is low, perhaps as
low as 97°; in the evening it is higher,
approaching, perhaps, 99°. It is the most
sensitive index of disease. A temperature
of 103° means definite fever; a temperature
of 106° means danger; a temperature of
109° usually means death. Temperatures
above and below " normal " are compatible
with life; but only for a time, and in particular diseases. If, with a temperature of
104°, whether the cause be known or not,
any individual follows his ordinary work, he
will probably die. Usually, such a temperature entirely disables him.

The pulse, the respiration, and the temperature, as a rule, vary together. Any one is
a provisional index to any other. They are
the most convenient normals for experimental
tests at the bedside. In a multitude of cases
they are all the physician needs to lead him
straight to the definite cause of the disorder.
Often, however, they are inadequate; and
then, even for the ends of immediate action,
he must proceed to a minute study of other
normals. To every shade and variety of the
" thousand ills," some normal function of

the body as a whole or of some special organ
definitely corresponds. To ascertain these
normals is the work of physiology ; to restore
any departure from them is the work of
curative medicine ; to prevent any departure from them is the work of preventive
medicine.

What, then, is a " normal " ? The action
of an organ varies within certain limits
without impairing the organ's elasticity or
structure.

In exercise, the heart may, in a few seconds,
rise from sixty beats a minute to one hundred
and twenty or more beats a minute. At the
end of the exercise, it returns in a few minutes
to the rate it started from. It suffers no
damage ; it retains its elasticity ; it maintains
its nutrition and its power of contraction.
Under the microscope, no fibre would be found
injured. It responds readily to every test.
And this is true of every normal heart. The
moment the elasticity is impaired or the
structure damaged, there is disease. If the
heart becomes " irritable," if palpitation
continues beyond an ascertainable average
of minutes, if excitement interferes with
the regularity of its beat, the exercise has
ended in disease.

For every organ of the body, there is a
similar average of function. For every group

of organs, there is an average of function.
For the body as a whole, there is a balance
of average functions. As the branch of a
tree sways this way and that in the wind
without losing the power to come back to
rest, so co-ordinated organs of the body vary
this way and that in response to the infinitely
varied needs of the environment, and yet
return uninjured to their co-ordinated balance.
And the body is an infinitely complex aggregation of growing structures. It is never at
rest. Of the millions of cells that compose
it, millions are dying every hour, millions
more are taking their places. But there is a
" moving equilibrium " of the whole. The
" moving equilibrium " has its index in an
average temperature, an average pulse, an
average respiration, average excretion, and a
thousand other averages that constitute the
special work of the anatomical, physiological,
and medical laboratories. Health is the
name we give to the total average of the
highest physiological efficiency. The organism
as a whole must maintain its place in the
struggle for life. It is by maintaining the
physiological normals that the organism maintains its place in the struggle. The maintenance of the physiological normals at their
highest potency is health. Any departure
from the normal that destroys the structure

of an organ or impairs its capacity to repeat its function is disease.

The objective signs of health are such as these,—readiness to act without external stimulus, capacity to act for prolonged periods without fatigue, regularity in the daily physiological cycles—cycles of appetite, cycles of muscular action, cycles of excretion, cycles of sleep. And there are many minor signs.

Subjectively, the healthy man has a feeling of satisfaction and ease in his activities, a general feeling of well-being, freedom from a sense of effort, freedom from the sense of environmental oppression, freedom from the feeling of being obsessed by his work, freedom from inner incontrollable moods or tempers. Every healthy man, in the dialect of his own philosophy, says—

> " God's in His heaven,
> All's right with the world."

CHAPTER II

THE CAUSES OF DEATH—THEIR NAMING AND CLASSIFICATION

LET us visit a Hospital for Sick Children and walk round with the surgeon.

Here are children of any age, from a few
months to fourteen or fifteen years. This,
the youngest, was born with club-foot, an
imperfect development that growth will never
by itself correct. An operation, at this stage
trivial, will prevent a lifelong disablement.
Another, somewhat older, suffers from knock-
knee. Now or at some later stage an operation, the brilliant invention of a great surgeon,
will straighten out the deformity. These
are defects rather than diseases. They are
not causes of death directly ; but indirectly
they may be causes of defeat in the race of
life. For they incapacitate the patient for
many occupations, and may lead him, in early
life, into neglect and destitution.

A third child, old enough to be at school,
has difficulty in breathing through the nose,
chokes in his sleep, and shows signs of defective nutrition. He suffers from enlarged
tonsils and adenoids (gland-like structures)
in the upper part of the throat. These he
will get removed by the surgeon, and forthwith
he will gain in weight and vigour. Another
has " bow-legs." His wrists and some other
joints are swollen. His ribs have curious
little knots in certain places. His chest
is somewhat misshapen. His head is un-
usually square and perhaps somewhat large
for his years. He suffers from rickets. The

disease has spontaneously stopped ; but the effects of it have remained and, unless partially corrected by surgery, will remain through life. He will grow into a strong man, but he may be somewhat deformed. His disease is a subtle and unexplained disease of nutrition, begun before his birth. His mother may have suffered from it ; but it is not necessarily an inherited disease. It may be due to food, or poisoning, or a failure of the organism to take in the correct quantity of lime from the food. Briefly, the cause is undetermined. But he is one of hundreds of thousands in the great cities. In one great city in Scotland, if you go where you can see poor children, you will find in half an hour a score of such cases.

Then observe the next bed. It is slightly tilted upwards ; it has a weight hanging over the end ; there is a child lying flat with a splint fixed along nearly the whole length of the body. This is a case of hip-joint disease, one of the innumerable forms of tuberculosis. Possibly, operation may be necessary if an abscess forms. Possibly, perfect rest may stop the mischief. In either case, the treatment will take months. In the next bed lies a case of spine disease,—another case of tuberculosis. In another case, it is the knee that is affected ; in another, the wrist ; and,

if you look farther along, it is the skin.   All
are tubercular.   Tuberculosis may affect any
organ in the body ; but the disabling effects
of it are most manifest when it appears in
the bones.   In the skin case, the form of
tuberculosis runs a slow, long course ; it has
been going on, perhaps, for five or ten years ;
it may end in death.   The name given to it
is *lupus*, probably because it seems to eat
away the tissue.   Fortunately, it can now be
cured, and the cure of it is one of the triumphs
of modern bacteriology.

Farther along lies a child with curiously
clouded eyes, sunken nose, and some other
deformities of the bones.   This is a case of
syphilitic infection.   His eyes are probably
damaged for life ; the destroyed bones will
never be restored ; other hidden destructions
may have taken place ; he may live for many
years, but he may never become a healthy
man.   This terribly merciless disease attacks
every organ of the body.   It can be cured,
but the cure often comes too late.

Let us now glance at a medical ward.   In
the first cot lies a child with lung disease—
possibly tuberculosis of the lungs, possibly
inflammation of the lungs (pneumonia), possibly bronchitis.   Its after-history of health
and fitness will depend much on which of the
three diseases it suffers from.   In other cots

lie cases of malnutrition, due, perhaps, to wrong feeding in early infancy, or to some defect in the digestive glands.   There are cases of bloodlessness, of rheumatism, of heart disease.

These are a few of " the causes of death " that a visitor may see at any time in a hospital for children.   The out-patient departments furnish masses of similar ailments ; some are less serious, but all are pulling the organism down.   Every disease is paid for by its own special form of unfitness.   No disease entirely passes.   After some diseases, definite disablements remain for life ;   of others, there are traces that impair vitality ; but of others, the effect is to adapt the organism better to its environment.   These, meanwhile, we may leave unvisited.   They are the acute infectious diseases.   As a rule, one attack protects a child against a second attack.

If you go to a general Hospital for Adults, you will find many of the same diseases still at work.   To maintain continuity of interest, let us imagine that the sick adults now to be seen are the same sick children ten, twenty, or thirty years older.   This is simpler than postponing our visit for ten or twenty years ; because, in so long a period, the names of

many diseases will change ; some of the
diseases will have lessened to vanishing
point ; new diseases or new ways of treating
them will have come to light.

On this occasion let us go round with the
physician.   The first case is a man who for
months has been wasting away for no reason
that can be discovered.   He suffers from
indigestion, but his trouble is not a digestive
disease.   He has lost flesh, energy, and interest.
He shows a marked pallor of countenance,
unusual depression, a strained and anxious
aspect.   He is probably suffering from some
malignant disease ; possibly cancer of the
stomach.   There are many such " malignant
tumours " ; there are many theories of their
origin ; but there is no explanation.   Almost
every pathological laboratory in the world
has some man searching for the cause of
malignant diseases.   A hundred times cures
have been announced, only to be a hundred
times discredited.   Such malignant tumours
may occur almost anywhere in the body,—
in the skin, in the lining of the stomach, in
the lining of the bowels, in the bones, in the
lungs, in the muscles, in the nerves, in the
brain.   There are many varieties, each taking
its character from the tissue of the part
affected ; but they are all malignant in
varying degrees.   They may be cut out ;

but they grow again. Occasionally, once
cut out, they never reappear. Occasionally,
too, when treated by the X-rays or Radium
they shrivel up and disappear. And there
are many instances where the growth is so
slow as almost to lose its character of malig-
nancy. When the cause and the cure of
cancer and the other malignant tumours are
discovered, mankind will be saved from a
great terror.

But note here a case of rheumatic fever—
a very acute illness, with high temperature,
rapid pulse, great pain in the joints, depression and helplessness. It often affects the
lining of the heart, external or internal ; so
producing imperfection of the heart valves
or disease of the external heart-lining, and
damaging the organ, perhaps, for the whole
lifetime. The disease is curable ; in some
degree, it is even preventable ; but it is one
of the most disabling, and, ultimately, one of
the most deadly, in the whole list. It may
recur several times, every time increasing
the damage. A heart so damaged may
partially recover ; it attains to a certain
plane of relatively healthy function ; it may
enable the man to follow his calling ; but it
will never permit him the same latitude of
physical labour, or exercise, or personal
exposure. Tens of thousands in the British

Islands are moving about with hearts once damaged by rheumatism. To this cause many of the sudden deaths are due. Any sudden exertion breaks down the partially restored heart and ends in greater disablement or in sudden death. Nor is this all. A heart so damaged may, through its intimate connections with the lungs and stomach, produce a chronic congestion of the breathing tubes, a chronic catarrh of the stomach, and possibly catarrh of the kidneys. Shortness of breath is a common symptom, because the damaged lung cannot do its work at the normal rate. If we followed up all the causes and consequences of rheumatic fever, we should have to describe diseases in many of the membranes and organs of the body.

Let us pass on to this case of lead poisoning. You notice that the patient cannot shake hands. He suffers from wrist-drop. His hand seems pulled in. This is because, at his trade as a painter, he has failed to keep his nails clean, or in some other way has succeeded in absorbing lead into the system. Lead affects the nerves that supply the hand, thus causing degeneration and paralysis. There are many other symptoms of chronic lead poisoning; but wrist-drop is the most striking. The disease is curable, if caught in time. It is, too, preventable, and ought not to occur. But it does occur in many occupations.

But who is this that is breathing so noisily ? He was picked up unconscious on the street ; his face very congested and somewhat drawn to one side. The physician tells us that a vessel in the brain has burst. This is apoplexy or cerebral hæmorrhage. When consciousness returns, he will find one arm or leg absolutely without power ; he can feel with them, but he cannot move them. And when he tries to speak, he will mumble and break his words. The clot in the brain due to the burst artery presses on the motor areas, interrupts the nerve paths from the brain to the limbs, and so produces paralysis. He will partially recover ; but he will never be the same man again. The causes of his ailment are various ; but the ailment itself will be classed as a disease of the nervous system.

In looking at the case of rheumatism, we have already seen diseases of the heart, which is the chief organ of the circulatory system. Here sits another case of heart disease. He suffers, at irregular intervals, from violent spasms of heart pain. He feels as if dying. When the spasm passes he is more or less exhausted, but, often, he is able to follow his duty. Sooner or later the spasms of pain will end in death. After death his heart will be found badly diseased; the valves of it may be found imperfect; the arteries that supplied it with nourishment will be found hard and inelastic. Near him is a man whose arteries are already far advanced in disease, hardened, robbed of their elasticity, ready to burst at any increase of pressure, slowing down the man's heart and with it his whole life. The condition, by care in early life, by the prevention of putrefaction in the bowels, by the careful adjustment of labour to capacity, by a judicious use of certain drugs, may be delayed and partially prevented; but, as we now see it, it is without remedy and may go on till the brain fails, producing senile imbecility and, one day, death.

Of diseases of the respiratory system there are many—pneumonia or inflammation of the lungs in several varieties, bronchitis, asthma, inflammation of the larnyx, not to speak of tuberculosis of the lungs, which, however, is an infectious disease, and will be studied more fully by itself. Many of the respiratory diseases are preventable; some of them being due to dust, some to a specific microbe; some to carelessness of clothing and exposure. Respiratory diseases account for the great mass of deaths.

There are, too, diseases of the digestive

system. Every organ of the alimentary
tract may furnish some disease that ends in
death. The mouth harbours many species
of infective germs ; some of them, it is said,
are the specific cause of a deadly form of
anæmia, and nearly all of them tend to produce one form or another of body poisoning.
The tonsils, apart from recurrent inflammation, may be the seat of scarlet fever, or
diphtheria, and may be an index of certain
rheumatic conditions. The stomach with
its many inflammatory and other diseases, the
bowels with their inflammations and ulcers,
the appendix with its many varieties of
appendicitis, the liver with its congestions,
or gall-stones, or tumours, or specific diseases,
the external lining of the bowels with its
inflammations, tubercular or other,—may all
provide causes of death.

It would take us a disproportionate time
even to name the classes of disease that yet
remain,—the diseases of the urinary system,
the diseases of pregnancy and child-birth,
the diseases of the skin, diseases of the
organs of locomotion, the diseases of early
infancy, not to mention the causes of death
by violence or accident. This, no less than
all that we have named, are to be found in
every large general hospital. They afford
endless material for the curative methods

both of the physician and of the surgeon.
There is not an organ of the body that may
not need skilled attention. And, if you
look at the ages marked on the bed-charts,
you will find that they vary from childhood
or adolescence to extreme old age. Every
stage of life has its predominating diseases,
but no stage is free from disease. Here,
the cause of disease is some poison like lead ;
there, it is over-exertion. Here, a disease
may come from improper feeding and in-
sufficient elimination of waste ; there, it
may come from under-feeding and inability
to withstand enforced exertion. This girl
is anæmic because she is confined in a lightless room all day, or lives on an ill-balanced
diet, or works among lead salts. That man
suffers from over-growth of the heart, because for years he has been over-worked and
under-fed. But of the causes of disease there
is no end. Every man and every organ he
possesses must respond in some way to the
environment if he is to live at all ; every
organ therefore has to meet, in due season,
its risks of over-pressure, of poisoning, or of
some other form of super-action or perverted
nutrition.

But it is not, for the moment, the causes
of disease we wish to emphasise. It is rather
that this chaos of activities, this unending

procession of diseases and defects, must have names, and must be classified. Otherwise, it would be impossible for science to master any of the causes of death.

Before searching for any principle to guide us in naming and classifying this chaotic mass of diseases, let us look for a moment into one hospital more—the Infirmary belonging to an English Workhouse or the Sick Wards of a Scottish Poorhouse. In these are collected the diseases of destitution, and the patients are a vast multitude. A glance proves that they have lived on a lower plane of health ; they are living now among more chronic diseases. Acute illnesses, like rheumatic fever, or appendicitis, are conspicuous by their rarity. Here the day is filled with the superabundance of old-standing heart disease, incurable paralysis of many varieties, incurable affections of the bones and joints, incurable blindness, incurable kidney disease, incurable results of syphilis, old leg-ulcers that need constant cleaning, running sores of bone that need constant dressing, the decrepitude of age, or the feeble-mindedness of youth, sometimes idiocy or imbecility in many grades and varieties, or epilepsy, or harmless forms of insanity, or disabling and incurable gout, or rheumatism, or brain disease, or spine disease, or some other of the thousand and one varieties of chronic disorder. There are, too, many malignant diseases, which are long beyond surgical or medical aid. All these diseases can be classified under the same heads as in the other hospitals ; but with a difference. The patients now visible are all on the waiting list for the grave. They drop off rapidly one by one : here, of senile feebleness ; there, of sudden heart failure or apoplexy. The men are old at fifty ; the women, senile. There is no green old age in the poorhouse. These are they that have dropped out of citizenship. They have lost touch with their fellows ; they live through the day without purpose, and when they die, they are buried by some one and their beds are filled again.

To widen our knowledge of the classes of disease, we ought to visit an Asylum for the Insane. A special field so vast would need a special list of names for the many diseases to be found there. The general word " insanity " covers a multitude of special diseases. Let us be content here to call them " mental diseases."

Nor shall we concern ourselves till later with the infectious diseases ; for they need special study.

How then shall we name and classify all

these departures from the normal, these palpable, visible, definable states of body ? The names come to us often with a long history ; many of them are derived from Latin or Greek ; but every one of them symbolises some state as clear to the physician and the surgeon as the eye or the hand is to the physiologist. But the kind of classification depends on the end to be served. It is said of a distinguished Aberdeen surgeon that, when he found something wrong with a knee-joint, he was content to say—" There is some infernal bobbery going on in that joint." This was fifty years ago. It was enough, in those days, to justify a surgical operation, and the surgeon achieved great things surgically. The science of diseased organs was then in its infancy. To-day the youngest surgeon that handles a knife knows in nine cases out of ten the precise nature of the condition he has to deal with, the course it will run if he does not operate, and the prospect of cure if he does. That he should be able to bring such knowledge to bear he owes largely to the fact that, for nearly sixty years, the causes of death have been carefully registered. In his reports weekly, monthly, quarterly, and yearly, the Registrar-General for each country places on record the numbers of those that die and the diseases that cause their death. To these reports every student of disease turns; from them he takes his data for the ends of medical, or surgical, or hygienic study, or for the purposes of insurance, or social research.

Since, however, the purposes of the classification are thus so various, the difficulties of satisfactory classification are enormous. Recently, under the leadership of France, an international Nomenclature of Diseases has been produced. This Nomenclature is the result of criticism and sifted experience. It has been adopted by some twenty nations or communities. It thus becomes an international code to facilitate the comparative study of disease and health. Not all diseases are here named; but all diseases are here provided with a class name. No departure from the normal will fail to find a general heading to suit it.

In this Nomenclature there are fourteen main blocks of disease. There are the general diseases, which include fifty-nine special classes; among these are all the infectious diseases, some thirty-two in all; the cancerous diseases; acute rheumatism; scurvy; diabetes; alcoholism, and other intoxications of various kinds. The second block includes the diseases of the nervous system and of the organs of sense. Then there are the

affections of the circulatory system; of
the respiratory system; of the digestive
system; of the genito-urinary system; the
puerperal state; the affections of the skin;
affections of the bones and organs of locomotion; imperfect developments and mon-
strosities; diseases of the new-born; diseases
of old age; diseases due to external causes,
such as violence; and a final class of badly
defined diseases. The sub-classes number
about one hundred and ninety. If each
morbid condition received a special name, the
list of names would far exceed a thousand.

What is the use of this elaborately sub-
divided Nomenclature of Diseases?   To
answer is easy. It enables the Doctor to
keep an exact record of the diseases he treats.
It enables him to enter in a death certificate,
as required by law, the primary and secondary
causes of death. It enables the local Regis-
trars all over the country to keep with exact-
ness the Register of Deaths for every locality.
It enables the Registrar-General to bring all
the facts for each cause of death into a single
Register. From the large numbers thus
collected, he is able to calculate the death-
rates due to each disease, to each group of
diseases, to each great class of diseases, to
the whole collection of diseases. From the
death-rates, he can infer the disease-rates of

every locality. He thus provides for the whole community an index of health. This index is the guide of all social progress. From it the individual citizen knows of the healthiness or unhealthiness of his village, or parish, or town, or city. From it the insurance companies draw data for their life-tables. From it the municipal world takes guidance in the cleaning of towns, in the reduction of overcrowding, in the rebuilding of unhealthy areas, and in the planning of cities. Without these sixty years of carefully calculated figures, the public health movement would be a movement in the dark. This is confirmed by the practice of every civilised country. No department of State activity can show greater justification than the department of statistics. The record of national health is the test of national progress.

It is for these reasons that so much detail is given here without apology. Every citizen should study national health records. He will gain from them a new significance for every form of social activity.

But the details given have a further purpose. They show the great dividing lines of disease. Each social organisation must choose for itself the divisions that suit its purpose ; but, in the study of health and disease, there is one fundamental division, namely, the division

between preventable and non-preventable
diseases. From our point of view, the progress of society is a progress from disease to
health. To prevent disease is to promote
health. But to prevent disease needs a knowledge not only of the methods of prevention,
but also of the diseases that are preventable.
Before, however, the significance of prevention can be understood, the death-rate must
be studied in somewhat greater detail.

CHAPTER III

DEATH-RATES AND THEIR INTERPRETATION

" IN the year 1908, the deaths from all
causes in England and Wales corresponded
to a rate of 14·683 per 1000 living at all ages
and of both sexes. This rate is the lowest
on record, and is below the average rate in
the five-year period ended 1907 by 5 per
cent."

What does this extremely condensed statement mean ? It is taken from The Seventy-
first Annual Report of the Registrar-General
for England and Wales. These figures, which

read so simply, represent a year's collection of facts in the provinces and months of calculation at the centre. The two sentences, therefore, deserve a careful analysis.

In the England and Wales of 1908, the deaths of 520,426 persons were registered. Of these, 268,714 were males and 251,742 were females. This is the first crude fact to be realised. It tells us little by itself; but nothing can be understood without it. Further, the population of England and Wales in the same year was not ascertained exactly, because 1908 was not a census year. On the basis, however, of the census of 1901, an estimate of the population was made. It was reckoned that, at the middle of 1908, the population amounted to 35,348,780, of whom 17,071,524 were males and 18,277,256 were females. This is the second crude fact to be realised. The population so ascertained was divided up among the various constituent areas,—towns, counties, and other administrative areas.

The rate, it is said, is the lowest on record. The record goes back to 1836. But it is enough to consider the facts of the last fifty years. For the five years from 1861 to 1865, the death-rate was equal to 21·4 per 1000 persons living. From that date, the Registrar-General reports, the death-rate fell

steadily, declining in the whole period under
review by nearly one-third. When, therefore, the rate is called " the lowest on record,"
it means that, for every thousand living,
only some fourteen die in each year as against
twenty-one fifty years ago.   There is thus a
saving of nearly seven lives for every thousand
of the population, and, as the population
numbered over 35 millions, the numbers saved
are enormous, being at least 245,000.   For
the ends of administration, the calculated
figure of 14·683 per 1000 symbolised all
this vast saving of life. But it is well,
occasionally, to translate back the rate into
the concrete facts and so make an effort to
realise in imagination the amount of life and
happiness the figures body forth for us.

But this death-rate of 14·6 per 1000 living
is not so simple as it seems.   It is a death·
rate of persons living " at all ages."   It,
therefore, in some way contains within
it the death-rates at each particular age.
If the population is analysed, it is found to
be made up of so many persons under five
years of age ; so many, from five to ten ;
so many, from ten to fifteen ; from fifteen
to twenty ; from twenty to twenty-five ;
from twenty-five to thirty-five ; from thirty-
five to forty-five ; from forty-five to fifty-
five ; from fifty-five to sixty-five ; from

sixty-five upwards. These are the ages
selected by the Registrar-General to parcel
out the population into convenient sections.
Each section has its predominant diseases,
its predominant causes of death, its own
current of sectional life. Children under
five, for example, tender, rapid-growing,
unstable, just entering the world of life's
stresses, infections, and injuries, naturally
have a higher death-rate than children of five
to ten, who have reached a relatively smooth
plane of life. At the other end of the scale
are the men and women over sixty-five.
They are past maturity ; they are living on
the remnants of their physiological capital ;
they are already " within the fore-shadows
of the tomb."

Imagine that, in the beginning of 1908, a
thousand children under five were placed in
the order of age from birth upwards and
certified living. If, at the end of 1908, the
same children were once more to be placed
in the same order, there would be forty
places unfilled. For, in that year, the death-
rate of children under five was 40 per 1000.
If, in the same year, a thousand persons over
sixty-five had been placed in their order,
the unfilled places at the end of the year
would have numbered eighty-seven. The
death-rate of persons over sixty-five was

87 per 1000.   Between these extremes there
are many variations.   The death-rate for the
children living between five and ten was 3
per 1000 ;   for children living between ten
and fifteen, it was nearly 2 per 1000 ;   and
for youths of both sexes living between
fifteen and twenty, nearly 3 per 1000 ;   for
those of twenty to twenty-five, over 3 per
1000 ;   for those of twenty-five to thirty-five,
nearly 5 per 1000 ;   for those of thirty-five
to forty-five, over 8 per 1000 ;   for those of
forty-five to fifty-five, over 14 per 1000 ;
for those of fifty-five to sixty-five, over 28
per 1000.

Has such an analysis any special value ?
It has immense value for many purposes.
It guides the student of health in his investigation of the conditions that foster disease.
It shows him what the feeble ages are, and
stimulates him to find the causes of enfeeblement.   It suggests many complicated questions for biology and sociology.   If our
population was formed solely of children aged
ten to fifteen, the death-rate would be less
than 2 per 1000.   If it were formed of men
and women over sixty-five, it would be nearly
90 per 1000.   In the urban counties it actually
was 94 per 1000 for those ages.   These death-
rates, therefore, suggest further analysis.   Obviously, if any community has a very large

proportion of children from ten to fifteen years old, its death-rate will be low. If it has a very large proportion of people over sixty-five, its death-rate will be high. The low death-rate of one locality, therefore, does not by itself prove that the locality is healthy, nor does the high death-rate of the other locality prove that it is unhealthy. It is clear that, if we are to compare the health of localities, the proportion of young and old in the population must be carefully esti-mated and allowed for. This is what is meant by " correction for age." There is a similar correction for the local differences in the relative numbers of males and females.

It would be possible to pass on from one fertile suggestion to another, until our minds were possessed with nothing but figures and the extraordinary revelations they bring. Figures are fascinating ; they are necessary ; they will never fail to attract the mathe-maticians and statisticians. But here we are concerned with other questions of practice. To us the death-rate is not an end in itself ; it is merely an index to what happens among our fellow-men, a guide to what can be done to remove the causes of death, an illuminating comment on the possibilities of preventing disease.

Look, then, for a moment at another aspect of the same facts. What are the most deadly diseases ? It is still the year 1908 that we study. The deaths from all causes were, as we saw, 520,426. If we took any thousand deaths, we should find that certain diseases contributed many more deaths than others. Thus, tuberculosis in all its forms contributed over 107 to every 1000 deaths—rather more than a tenth of the whole. Tuberculosis of the lungs alone contributed 76 to the 1000 deaths. In the list of contributors, tuberculosis is an easy first. Next come diseases of the heart, which contributed 96 to the 1000 deaths. Then follow diseases of the respiratory system, with a contribution of 89 per 1000 deaths. If pneumonia, which is now classified as an infection, were added, the total contribution of respiratory diseases would be nearly 170. Diseases of the nervous system contributed 64 ; cancer and other malignant diseases, 63 ; old age, 63 ; diseases of the blood-vessels, 60 ; diseases of the digestive system, 55. The most fatal infections of that year were measles, contributing 15 ; influenza, contributing 19 ; whooping-cough, contributing 19 ; diphtheria, contributing 11 ; diarrhœa, contributing 35,—to every 1000 deaths.

One clear impression emerges—the great

death-dealing diseases are tuberculosis, diseases of the heart and blood-vessels, and diseases of the respiratory system. The others all are important, but no single group can rival these. It is now clear why, in our visits to the hospitals, these great diseases were found in the ascendant. Wherever we went, we encountered them. At that stage, they were diseases of the living, claiming sympathy and skill; at this stage, they are causes of death, recorded in the cold quantities of administrative science.

But this analysis of a thousand deaths concerns only a single year, and a total death-rate of 14·6 per 1000 living. It is the progress of the death-rate year by year that tells us where we are going. Let us look backwards. This time our illustration may come from Scotland. The diseases on record there are just the same and tell the same story.

Of two diseases, the history is marvellous—typhus fever and smallpox. It was not till the year 1865 that typhus fever and typhoid (enteric) fever were separately recorded. Indeed, only a short time before then were they definitely known to be distinct. They are still occasionally confused; but, in the typical cases, no confusion is possible. It may be assumed, however, that of the two, typhus contributed more than typhoid to the enormous total of deaths. In 1855 the Scottish deaths from these two diseases numbered 2419, representing a death-rate of 90 for every 100,000 of the population. The deaths fell a little and rose a little in the ten years; but in 1864 the two diseases together killed 4804 people, corresponding to a death-rate of 116 for every 100,000 of the population. In 1865 the deaths from each disease were separately recorded. In that year typhus alone killed 3272—a death-rate of 108 per 100,000.

Mark now the change. In 1880 typhus killed only 170 people—a death-rate of 5 per 100,000. In 1890 it killed only 77—a death-rate of 2 per 100,000. In 1900 it killed only 35 people—a death-rate of 1 per 100,000. In 1908 it killed eight persons—a fractional rate per 100,000. Consider the average rates for the ten-yearly periods—91 (the two diseases), 65, 15, 3, 1, less than 1, per 100,000. A disease that alone numbered tens of thousands of sick and its thousands of dead has practically vanished in fifty years. It is so rare that, when it comes, it is usually taken for something else. But it is so virulent that it always compels attention. The extirpation of this disease is a triumph

of administration. It is a supreme example
of what can be done by isolation, uncrovding,
drainage, cleansing, and the systematic removal of waste. The germ that causes the
disease is still undiscovered ; but the natural
history of the disease is well understood.
The tale told of Scotland is true of England
and Ireland. Once, typhus was a scourge in
Europe ; to-day, it is hardly to be found
among the causes of death.

The history of smallpox is little less striking.
If, again, ten-yearly periods are taken, the
smallpox death-rates are these—35, 18, 19, 1,
per 100,000.

For scarlet fever the corresponding figures
are 98, 96, 79, 29, 19, per 100,000. There
is here a steady fall in the death-rate. After
typhus and smallpox, scarlet fever has
received the lion's share of administrative
attention. The death-rate from it everywhere
has gone down ; but the disease still comes
back in frequent epidemics ; it always rises in
the autumn and tails off in the spring ; but
it is universally allowed to be a less serious and
more manageable disease than it was thirty
or forty years ago. But measles, which from
the average of the five years after 1855
killed 43 per 100,000, still continues its ravages
almost unchecked ; for, on the average of the
ten years after 1891, it killed 47 per 100,000.

With one depressing fact, this chapter must end. The death-rate from cancer and other malignant diseases was, on the average of the ten years following 1861, 42 per 100,000. The average of the ten years following 1891 was 74 per 100,000. Allow for improved diagnosis—which is the fact ; allow for the great saving of life up to the cancer ages— which is also the fact ; allow, too, that the increase has not occurred in the easily accessible and readily recognisable cancers, as of the lip, the tongue, the face, but rather in the hidden cancers of the internal organs. It matters little. The dreary, depressing fact remains. Up till now cancer must be labelled " incurable." But the scientific passion of the world is centred on it in a hundred laboratories. Already, hints of discovery are everywhere ; for all we know, perhaps the discovery is already made. The history of other diseases allows us to hope ; for scientific pathology is not a century old. Possibly within the lifetime of the middle-aged, cancer will pass into the class of preventable diseases.

CHAPTER IV

FEVER, INFECTIOUS DISEASE, AND EPIDEMICS

In 1844, the Commissioners appointed to inquire into the administration and practical operation of the Poor Law in Scotland issued their report. Among other things, they reported on the problems of medical relief to the poor. In particular, they reported on " fever " and epidemics, which, in those days, were recorded as inevitable incidents of individual and social life. Typhus was everywhere. Smallpox was everywhere. In one town of Western Scotland a careful schoolmaster and session-clerk divided the people into two classes—those that had taken smallpox and those still to take it ! Of the infections now most common—scarlet fever, measles, and whooping-cough—less is heard. They were probably masked by typhus, smallpox, and enteric fever. They were all well known ; but they were of less account than the great death-dealers.

It is in such a social atmosphere that the Commissioners of 1844 write in reference to fever and epidemics: " It is, however, very questionable whether the periodical prevalence of fever in these places—that is, in Edinburgh and Glasgow—can justly be ascribed to any specific cause. There may be said to be three distinct opinions on the subject. The first is stated in the Sanitary Report, it attributes the spread of fever to filth and defective sewerage ; the second would ascribe the evil to an overcrowded population ; the third, to destitution. We believe it to be true that wherever fever prevails, one or more of these concomitants will be found to exist. But as to the amount of influence which all or any of such causes may have on the diffusion or origin of disease, we feel that it would be presumptuous in us to offer any opinions, where medical men of the greatest experience are not agreed."

In those days it was not possible to be more exact. The infectivity of certain fevers was well known ; but the germ theory had not yet come to light. There was no science of bacteriology. Not for some years after 1844 did it enter the mind of any investigator to suggest a bacillus or any other microbe as the cause of enteric fever, or diphtheria, or smallpox, or typhus, or measles. Indeed, for several of these diseases no germ has yet been isolated ; but analogy leaves us in little doubt that for them all a specific germ will be found. In those days, too, there was little effort at sanitation. The reports of

Chadwick and Neil Arnot on the state of Glasgow are sad reading. Except in the more remote and most neglected hamlets or villages of to-day, the lower animals are housed in better conditions than in those days the human beings were. The fevers were lumped together under the vague name of " fever." In medicine, the word is now the name of a symptom—the rise of temperature above the normal. But, used of an un-differentiated mass of virulent sicknesses, it acquired a terrible meaning, whose traditions you find still living in the popular mind.

It is difficult to understand why, even at that date, the distinction of infectious types was so little advanced. The great physicians knew them well ; for their descriptions are extant. Perhaps the lesser medical men had little chance of attaining to even such science as existed. It is certain that the study of infection had not advanced far ; for, at the beginning of the century, a distinguished physician is still proving the infectivity of whooping-cough. The want of scientific methods of research accounts for much, and seventy years ago the physician had not grasped the conception of prevention. He looked on " fevers " much as more recently he looked on " tropical diseases,"—that is, as a chaos without a clue. It is probable that

" fever " included diseases as diverse as these — typhus fever, typhoid fever, pneumonia, cerebro - spinal fever, tubercular meningitis (inflammation of the brain membranes), appendicitis, septicæmia (blood-poisoning), and some others. But, in spite of their inadequate knowledge, the Commissioners of 1844 made many recommendations of a fruitful kind and prepared the way for the public health services we now enjoy.

To point the differences between then and now, let us visit a modern Public Health Hospital of one hundred beds. It is built in six separate pavilions. It has an administration block standing apart. Between each two pavilions there is a clear space, forty feet wide. There are a laundry and disinfecting block, a discharging block, and all the other offices needed for the management. The whole is spread over some five or six acres. It is really a group of separate hospitals ; for each pavilion houses but a single disease, and, at the moment, there are perhaps four or five or six diseases, and the whole six pavilions are in full occupation. Each patient has 2000 cubic feet of room. It will, therefore, be easy to see how the " fever " of the old days is now split up in order that it may be conquered.

In the first block, where scarlet fever is housed, there are a score of children, varying in age from two upwards ; possibly one or two adults. It is a fair index of the proportional incidence of the disease. Here is a school child of ten, just admitted. His face is flushed, but there is no " rash " on it. His hands, arms, chest, body, and lower limbs, however, all show a bright red eruption,— the rash of scarlet fever. He has some difficulty with his breathing ; for his throat is much inflamed and his tonsils swollen. His eyes, too, are congested. He is excited, but feeble. His pulse runs at a high rate. His temperature has gone up to 103° F. or 104° F. It will remain near that figure for a day or two. The rash will fade away in forty-eight hours. The throat will grow less painful. Any discharge from the nose will diminish. The pulse will slow down. In perhaps four days he will be back, apparently, to his normal state. A new process, however, begins. The skin, formerly so bright red, is now pale and dry. Within a week, sometimes much earlier, sometimes later, it begins to be shed. The shedding goes on until the face, neck, body, arms, legs, and even the hands and feet are completely cleared of the old skin. The process may take weeks. Through all this period the patient is ex-

tremely susceptible to cold.   He may develop
complications ;   the kidneys may become
inflamed, and death from dropsy may result.
But, if all goes well, he is out of bed, out of
ward, and out of hospital well within six, seven,
or eight weeks.

Every year tens of thousands of British
children run through this history.   They die
at the rate of some 3 per cent. of all those
affected.   In the old days, the death-rate was
higher ; but we are not certain whether the
disease was quite the same.   Possibly it was
" a mixed infection " ; as typhus and typhoid
were rolled into one, so possibly scarlet fever
and some other virulent infection went
together.   In modern days, severe cases
frequently occur ; but, for the most part, the
cases are mild.

You ask how this child was infected.
Possibly, he drank infected milk.   Possibly,
he caught directly the infective discharge
of some other patient ; but whatever the
immediate origin, there is always " the one
before."   From thirty-six hours to three, four,
or five days after he " catches " the infection, he shows the symptoms in the sequence
described.

We pass now to the typhoid pavilion.
Three weeks ago this woman was nursing a

case of known typhoid fever.   A week ago
she began to suffer from bad headache ; her
temperature began to rise ; in three days it
had reached 104° F.   She is now at the end of
the first week after the onset of the disease,
the invasion.   The temperature remains high,
falling a little in the morning, rising again at
night.   For three weeks it will continue so.
Gradually, while maintaining the same vibra-
tions night and morning, it will on the whole
slowly subside, until in the fourth week it will
be once more normal.   Meanwhile, the patient
suffers little pain, but great prostration.   She
has to be kept on a rigidly limited diet ;
because the bowels are ulcerated and much
food might be dangerous.

The disease is due to a specific germ, which
may be swallowed with milk, or water, or food,
and must have come from a previous case.
Within six weeks of the onset of the illness,
this woman will be well, but profoundly
feeble.   Mentally, she may suffer for a time ;
for delirium is a common symptom of the
disease, and it may be followed by temporary
feebleness of mind.   In France, typhoid fever
is looked upon with much alarm ; for it is a
common starting-point of functional nervous
diseases.   Any shock, or fright, in the period
of feebleness may, without the after knowledge
of the patient, result in serious nervous

disturbances that may affect the whole after life. These results are not common in this country; but they indicate the need for careful nursing and the greatest attainable quietness and peace.

But there may be another result. The patient herself may recover; but she may continue to be infectious. In her excretions the bacillus of typhoid fever may remain active for weeks, for months, for years. In a word, she may become " a carrier case." Immune to the disease herself, she will remain capable of infecting others. She will harbour in the liver (in the gall-bladder) an innumerable host of typhoid germs. From time to time these will pass into the blood or the bowel and afterwards be diffused just as if she still suffered from the disease.

It is only some five years ago since this condition was thoroughly understood. At a certain Continental restaurant every new servant that came took typhoid fever. There was nothing in the water, in the milk, in the food, in the sanitation of the house to account for the occurrences; but the head of the establishment had some years before suffered from typhoid. She was still infectious. The case was carefully studied, and scores upon scores of such cases are now on record.

The carrier case accounts for many apparently unaccountable outbreaks of typhoid fever. Murchison, the greatest English authority on typhoid and typhus, held a theory that typhoid fever could originate from uninfected filth. In the days before bacteriology, such a theory was justifiable provisionally; now that the germ and the carrier case are known, the hypothesis is superfluous. The carrier case presents very difficult administrative problems; but the experts are busy at research, and the prospects of a radical cure are already promising.

Incidentally, let it be said that the carrier case is not confined to typhoid fever. It may occur in scarlet fever, in diphtheria, in cerebro-spinal fever, in tuberculosis, and possibly in several other infections. In all those named, such cases have been demonstrated. Patients that recover from those diseases may carry germs with them and hand them on to infect others. But it is not even necessary that the carrier should himself have had the disease. He may have caught the germ from another; he may carry it about with him, growing in his nose or throat, harmlessly; he may hand it on to a third person, and so maintain the continuity of the disease. This gives a new significance to the " contacts "—the persons exposed to infection. Of these, some are perhaps immune to the given infection, but they are capable of cultivating the germ on their tissues. Others may catch the disease and remain infectious. Yet others are incapable either of catching the disease or maintaining the germ of it alive. But all three classes must be dealt with if the radiations of the disease are to be stopped.

From these we might pass to the measles cases, or the chickenpox cases, or the cerebrospinal cases, or the mixed infections like scarlet fever and diphtheria, or scarlet fever and chickenpox, or measles and scarlet fever. But we have already seen sufficient to give us the type of an infectious fever.

It so happens, however, that there is typhus in hospital to-day. Typhus now comes only in little outbreaks. It is an infection easily killed. It never goes far. Here is a group of severe cases, of whom the forerunner was a supposed case of pneumonia. The two diseases are totally distinct, but they resemble each other in some symptoms. Sometimes they are concurrent. In this outbreak the supposed pneumonia must have been typhus. The patients lie on their back ; muttering to themselves ; picking at the bedclothes ; faces flushed ; eyes closed ; heedless ; helpless. There is an eruption of very characteristic type. There is, too, an offensive odour. The patients will lie in the same attitude for days on end.

Here is one on the fourth day of her illness. Some twelve or thirteen days before the invasion began, her brother had died of supposed pneumonia. Her temperature ran rapidly up to 104° F. or 105° F., and has kept near that level for the four days. If she lives, the temperature will continue high until the thirteenth or fourteenth day, when it will drop in a few hours to normal. Every symptom will have disappeared, and the delirious, oblivious patient will come to herself, clear-minded and smiling.

This sudden transformation I have seen many times. The whole violent invasion ends as rapidly as it began. It is a raid of microbes. Too often it destroys the life. Children sleep through it peacefully ; the middle-aged and the old mostly die. With the exception of smallpox, the disease is probably the most infectious of all infections known to the West. Repeatedly, it has been suggested that it is transferred by fleas. It will strike through the air at as great a distance as a flea jumps. It is certain that, whatever the virus be, it does not live long in the air. The flea hypothesis needs proving ; but it has much in its favour.

Typhus, I have said, is often mistaken for some other disease. I have seen it mistaken for the following : influenza, meningitis, pneumonia, typhoid fever, bronchitis. No disease vanishes more rapidly under preventive measures ; but the swiftness of its spread, the difficulty of recognising it, its origin in filth, squalor, overcrowding, and destitution all make it somewhat difficult to handle administratively. And the danger to life is great. Unlike smallpox, it cannot be warded off by vaccination. Unlike typhoid, it spreads swiftly by the air, whether carried by fleas or not. Unlike diphtheria, it is not located in any special part of the body ; it is a diffused infection. But, as we have seen, it has vanished from its place at the head of fatal epidemic diseases, and now recurs here and there, to remind us that there are slums in town and county still to be destroyed.

Fevers, it is now seen, have been parcelled out into perfectly definite classes. From these classes some inferences are possible. The infectious fevers are no longer a shapeless mass of unexplained signs and symptoms ; they are a group of specific diseases. Each of them has a natural history of its own. Each of them can be tracked separately along its whole course. Each of them is treated in

the ways adapted to its habits.   But, separate
and specific though they are, these diseases
have certain common features.   These it is
important to know ; for they are the general
guide both to theory and to administration.

The infective agent always comes from
without.   It may be a minute rod-shaped
plant (bacillus), as in diphtheria ; or an
organism of higher grade, as in malaria ; or
a form unknown, as in smallpox, typhus,
scarlet fever, measles, chickenpox, and many
others.   That in every case it is an organism
with a life-history of its own, there is no
reasonable doubt.   The science of bacteriology
is still young ; but it has discovered hundreds
of unsuspected germs,—unveiling their life-
histories by observation and experiment, and
proving whether they are disease-producers or
not.   Though but partially verified, the germ
theory may be accepted at least provisionally.   The diseases, like smallpox, whose
germ is yet unrevealed, behave precisely
like those whose germ is known.   But, germ
or no germ, the general features of infection
are always the same.

The infective agent, then, always comes from
without.   It may be breathed in with the
dust, as probably in smallpox.   It may be
swallowed with water, as often in enteric
fever.   It may be swallowed with milk, as

often in enteric fever, scarlet fever, diphtheria,
and tuberculosis. It may enter the blood
through a scratch in the skin, as in anthrax,
or in blood-poisoning from a pricked finger.
It may be injected by a flea, as probably in
plague. It may be injected by a mosquito,
as certainly in malaria and yellow fever. It
may be growing for months or years in the
mouth, as probably the pneumococcus does ;
for Professor Osler, in a vast number of
examinations, found the pneumococcus
present in practically every mouth examined
except the mouths of the tobacco-chewing
negroes. Or again, the infective agent may lie
harmless for a period in the nose, as probably
in cerebro-spinal fever and possibly in erysipelas. Sometimes the infective agent enters
by one channel, sometimes by another, even
in the same disease.

The channels of infection are a profoundly
difficult problem in pathology. No subject
excites more interest at medical conferences ;
none creates a more acute division of opinion.
Is the germ of tuberculosis breathed into the
lungs, and does it start its nefarious course
there ? Or is it swallowed with the dust,
entering the blood - stream through the
bowels ? The practical consequences are far
from unimportant. If it enters directly
into the lungs, the time of its reappearance

in the material coughed up has one meaning,—the presence of the germ would be
an early symptom. If it enters indirectly
through the bowel, passing by the lymphatic
channels into the blood-stream and ending in
the lungs, its reappearance in the material
coughed up would have another meaning,—
the presence of the germ would be a late
symptom. And so with endless variations
for each of the infections. For years to
come, the precise channel of entrance for
many diseases will remain a problem. In
plague, for instance, one of the most difficult
parts of the late Royal Commission's work was
the determination of the channel of entry.
It is fascinatingly simple to assume that,
as millions of Indian natives go bare-footed,
the rat fleas would most readily attack the
lower limbs, and the buboes of plague would
most frequently appear in the groin. But
this solution is almost too easy. How
complex the problem is any one may learn
from the pages of the Commission's Report.
Sir Thomas Fraser's analysis of the anatomy
of the lymphatic glands or lymphatic vessels
is a classic piece of applied science. It shows
how many factors enter into a problem
apparently simple. The general drift of
recent information is that the rat flea does
convey plague from the rat to man ; that it

does inoculate the lymphatics, and that a proportion of the innumerable cases is due to this cause. We leave the question open; it will soon be closed by the evidence now accumulating. Already, the evidence is enough to require that every precaution shall be taken against rat fleas and rats.

Volumes have been written on the channels of infection. Here we are concerned only with illustrations. But it is definitely proved that malaria is spread by a particular species of mosquito and by no other means; that yellow fever is spread by another form of mosquito, and by no other means; that flies, on their feet, may convey typhoid and other germs for long distances; that rat fleas can convey plague from rat to rat, and almost certainly from rat to man; that many species of tropical insects can inoculate the human body with deadly diseases. The massed details of the splendid researches that justify these conclusions have opened up for us an illimitable field for further investigation. To biology preventive medicine owes as much as to the study of disease at the bedside.

The infective agent, once it enters the body, seems for a time to lie dormant. This

is its incubation period. The incubation
may last only a few hours, as occasionally in
scarlet fever. It may last for twelve or
thirteen days, as in typhus fever, or measles,
or smallpox. It may last for twenty-one
days, as in mumps, and, occasionally, in
typhoid fever. It may last for four, five,
or six weeks, as in syphilis. It may last
for a period unknown, as in hydrophobia.
Even in the same disease, it varies from a few
hours to several days, as in scarlet fever,
where, however, it practically never exceeds
five days.

In diseases like pneumonia, or diphtheria,
it is difficult to give a precise meaning
to the term incubation. For, in those
infections, the germ may grow in the
mouth or in the tonsils for weeks or
months without producing a single per-
ceptible symptom. In tuberculosis, too, the
germ may go on growing in the tissues of
the body for years without producing one
sign discoverable by naked-eye observation.
And the term incubation does not seem to
fit well to the history of a recurrent fever
like malaria. There, the infective agent at
once enters the blood-stream, affects the
blood corpuscles, running through a series of
changes that end in fever, and then again in
a period of quiescence. The process comes

and goes in ascertainable periods.   But for
none of the periods does the term incubation
seem suitable.

The infective agent, I have said, seems to
lie dormant.   But it is only " seems."
Perhaps it is growing, as in a laboratory
incubator, until it has amassed numbers
sufficient to make an attack in force.   Possibly this occurs in diphtheria, where the
germ may often be found in masses on the
surface of the tonsil.   Or, perhaps, it is
actively breaking down the natural defences
offered by the blood cells, the blood liquids,
the tissue cells and the tissue liquids.   These
all probably contain or produce antidotes
to those living poisons.   Once the antidotes
are all exhausted, then the germ may advance freely, conquering and to conquer.
It may increase in numbers until the dose of
its poison overwhelms millions of the body
cells.   Then, indeed, the incubation is over ;
but is incubation the best name for this war
between two species ?

Or, once more, the infective germ, having
lost its virulence in passing through another
body, may need nursing and nourishment
before it can deal a blow at a new enemy.
Or, yet again, it may enter a body where
it is biologically welcome, or not exceptionally unwelcome.   In a group of

smallpox cases, all in one family, I have
seen every grade of infection from a single
doubtful spot on the skin of the youngest
child, to a well-marked eruption on an
older sister. Between the two extremes
lay other cases that showed what the extremes meant. In one case appeared an
eruption that seemed to be the forerunner
of a violent confluent smallpox ; but in
forty-eight hours this eruption disappeared.
In another, some thirty trifling pocks formed
and slowly disappeared,—a modified smallpox. Is incubation the name for the process that had an issue in each case so different ?
Surely not. Probably the incubation period
covers a various multitude of active processes,
each peculiar to the given disease. It may
even be that the germ is actively immunising
against itself the whole tissues of the body,
and that the final outburst that we name " the
disease," the " fever," is only a too rapid, too
violent process of immunisation.

These are some of the puzzles that cluster
round the incubation period. They are a
type of innumerable problems that have
sprung up since the germ theory appeared.
They complicate the study of medicine ; but
they show how intricate the adaptations of
the body are to the infinitely various environment. But the increasing application of

theories does on the whole result in an increasing simplification of practice.

Let us pass on. When the incubation is over, the invasion begins. The temperature rises, there is shivering, distress, perhaps vomiting, perhaps even convulsions. In a time that varies from an hour or two to three days or more, the invasion is complete. The temperature remains at a certain level; the pulse and the respiration keep company with it.

Perhaps the invasion means, as I have said, the beginning of the last stage of the war. It is different in each disease. In typhoid fever, it is shown perhaps only by a headache. In smallpox, it often begins with pain in the back. In diphtheria, it often starts with sudden prostration. In scarlet fever of infants, it may produce convulsions. In practically every disease, it is something violent and striking, even to the most casual observer. With the invasion, too, begins, as a rule, the period of active infectivity. Before the invasion the infected person is not himself infectious. You can eat with him, and drink with him; but you will not catch infection from him. After the invasion, it is entirely different; he is a danger to his fellows. It is then that he

invokes the public health service. In ignorance, he may have caught the infection;
but after the invasion, he remains in ignorance
no more; he is sick physically and mentally.
Like a man intoxicated, he finds his ideas in
confusion, his will overpowered, his feelings
beyond his control. He is glad to have done
with action and thinking; he is content to
leave himself to the care of his friends.

Once the invasion is over, the patient runs
a more or less level course for times that
vary with each disease. If he has lost consciousness, he occasionally, for short periods,
recovers it. If he has not lost consciousness,
he establishes a sort of relative health on the
new plane. If the disease goes favourably,
he gradually regains the mastery of himself.
Sometimes he suddenly drops to normal;
sometimes he glides into it imperceptibly, like
an alighting bird. The fight between the
infective agents and the tissues is done, and
the victory is with the greater organism.
The danger to himself is over; but the
danger to his fellows is not. If the disease has
been smallpox, the infective agent reappears
in the gross, palpable eruption, which forms
large scabs on the skin. The scabs dry and
crumble into dust. The dust passes into the
air, or is scattered over the room, or is caught

in the clothing, or adheres to utensils. In a hundred ways, it is spread abroad once more. Every grain contains fresh infective material. So long as a scab remains on the skin the patient remains a danger. But the day comes when all the scab drops off, when the skin can be finally disinfected, when the patient may with safety resume his place in the ranks of society. And so it is with nearly every infection. Through all the time of its activity there is danger. But each disease, as it had a definite beginning, has a definite end. The infective agent comes in, fights with the forces against it, and at the end passes out—perhaps in greater multitudes, but almost always for ever.

And that leads to an important truth,—some infections infect only once and never again. This knowledge is as ancient as history. The explanation of it is still to find. Of the fact, however, there is no doubt. Take smallpox once and you will not take it again—or almost certainly not; for there are known exceptions. Take scarlet fever and you will probably not take it again. Take measles and you will probably not take it again. Take chickenpox and you will almost certainly not take it again. Is this true also of diphtheria, or enteric fever, or typhus, or malaria, or plague ? It is not true absolutely, but it is partly true. In most of those diseases, one attack absolutely protects against another for a varying time. The conditions of protection are not yet completely investigated. The problem is among the most difficult in the whole range of biology.

The theories of protection or immunity are not merely fascinating ; they are of great practical importance. They deserve our attention. For, if one thing marks more distinctively than another the research of the present generation, it is the effort to discover the conditions of immunity. The fact is old ; the methods of investigating it are young. Inoculation with mild smallpox to forestall severe smallpox is a custom centuries old. Vaccination is more recent, but the fundamental idea is the same. To these theories we return later.

In one of the Acts of Parliament, diseases are divided into epidemic, endemic, or infectious diseases. The division is not logical ; but it is convenient. When a disease foreign to the country, or non-existent at the time in any community, enters and spreads among the people, it is called epidemic. The word is also loosely used to describe any large outbreak of disease, infectious or other. When a disease propagates itself within an area, persisting there indefinitely, affecting person after person, it is called endemic.   Up till late in the nineteenth century, malaria was endemic in England ; tuberculosis is endemic now.   These terms are in common use ; and the legal application of them has had great practical consequences.

Under certain powers the Local Government Board can impose certain far-reaching obligations upon the local health authorities— notification of disease, house to house visitation, rapid burial of the dead, provision for hospital accommodation, supply of medicines and treatment, and any other duties necessary to prevent the spread of the disease.   These powers are of immense value internationally ; for, as will be shown later, they constitute our chief protection against the importation of plague, cholera, and yellow fever.   Nationally, to judge by the recent Tuberculosis Orders of the English Local Government Board, they promise to become a potent factor in the prevention of our great endemics.

To illustrate compactly an epidemic of infection is difficult ; for the conditions of its actual occurrence are so complex that the details are apt to interest only the individual officer.   But the general course of an epidemic may be represented by a curve. Assume that a scarlet fever patient moves about uncontrolled. He meets in every relation of society some people susceptible to the disease. He thus infects several, who in turn infect others. As time goes on, the numbers infected increase ; the curve rapidly or slowly rises. A time—weeks, months, years —comes when all the susceptible people in a community have contracted the infection. Gradually, the curve declines, and at last again reaches the level. If the death-rate alone, not the disease-rate, be taken as the index, the curve will also, periodically, rise into similar epidemic peaks. When the epidemic is over, another crop of susceptible people begins to grow. When their number reaches a certain ratio to the whole population, there is apt to be another explosion.

In a milk epidemic, the course is some-what different. Instead of spreading from person to person, the disease spreads suddenly in the milk. Twenties and thirties may be infected in a single day. These tend to start sub-epidemics among their contacts, and so we have a compound epidemic. In water epidemics, it is the same ; the outbreak is sudden, and it ends rapidly when the water is withdrawn or sterilised. Milk and water epidemics resemble wholesale poisonings of the susceptibles rather than infection from person to person.

But, generally, an epidemic follows one type,—sudden appearance of infection from beyond the borders of the community; a series of severe illnesses linked one to the other or to a common source; a sudden cessation of the epidemic when the source is discovered and countered by appropriate measures; some deaths; many survivals, protected for years or for life.

Endemic infectious diseases tend to rise, from time to time, into epidemics. Scarlet fever, at its lowest in April, rises steadily to November and then declines. Enteric fever, at its lowest from May to July, rises to November and similarly declines. Measles, at its lowest in February, rises above its normal in June, falls to its lowest in September, and reaches its climax in December, declining again in February. Whooping-cough rises in January, to a climax in March and April, falls to a minimum in September and October, and then rises again. The course of smallpox is somewhat the same. Diarrhœa reaches its maximum in July.

These seasonal variations may be complicated by the conditions of industry, aggregation in schools, the activity of the preventive authorities, and other incidental factors.

But the rises and falls with the seasons show how each disease follows its own natural history.

If you wish to study epidemics in detail, as they are managed by the sanitary authorities of England, procure the reports of the medical inspectors of the Local Government Board. These, in a series extending over many years, illustrate, in endless variety, the methods of preventive medicine in dealing with disease and its causes. Studies on a larger scale are to be found in the reports by the medical officer of the Board. Unfortunately, there is no difficulty in obtaining accounts of actual epidemics ; for the reports by the medical officers of health of town and county have still to record scores upon scores of outbreaks every year. And reports by the medical inspectors of schools add to our materials, already too great.

Biologically, it fascinates the observer to study the fight between the minor organism and the major ; administratively, it often exhausts the medical officer of health to dissociate the combatants. But, as time goes on, the biologist becomes more of a medical officer and the medical officer more of a biologist.

CHAPTER V

STUDY OF A TOXIC INFECTION AND ITS ANTITOXIN

WHAT is diphtheria ?

For Biology, it is an incident in the life-history of a micro-organism—the Klebs-Löffler bacillus—during its residence in a human or other animal body.

For Chemistry, it is a means of generating two, if not three, kinds of poison—one kind a ferment, another an albumose (allied to albumen or white of egg), and the third an organic acid.

For Pathology, it is a sequence of tissue-changes, beginning usually in the throat and ending in the muscles, nerves, or other structures ; so causing nerve-degenerations, muscle-degenerations, local and general paralyses ; these conditions being the result of the poisons manufactured by the Klebs-Löffler bacillus.

For the Practice of Medicine, diphtheria is a disease of the throat, very frequently fatal, most frequently fatal in children under five, running an indefinite course, liable to recur, frequently attended by complications ; affecting both the local organs and the general constitution, sudden in onset, treacherous in results, sometimes as easy to treat as a bleeding finger, at other times baffling every resource of the most skilful.

For Hygienics or Public Health, diphtheria is a highly infectious disease, liable to spread chiefly by personal contact; varying with the yearly rainfall; apt to become epidemic after a series of dry seasons; not demonstrably connected with bad drains or bad water, but frequently with low-lying and damp houses; capable of being carried by milk, by clothing, by dust, by cats, by cows; sometimes associated with crowding in schools; always capable of being confined by isolation.

The precise scientific knowledge of diphtheria is essential to an intelligent campaign for its prevention. I propose, therefore, to order my remarks according to the sciences I have named. Our study will thus be at once theoretical and practical, a synthesis of science and administration. But first I shall steady our minds by a short account of a concrete case. It occurred sixteen years ago, when antitoxin was still a new drug on its trial, not the seasoned friend it has since become.

One morning a medical practitioner, as required by the Infectious Disease Notification Act, intimated at my office a case of diphtheria. He had that morning, at seven o'clock, been summoned to a girl of eight. He found her suffering from great difficulty of breathing (croupy symptoms), pallor of the face, blueness of the lips, subnormal temperature, feeble pulse. She had been ill for a day or two at least. Emergency remedies rallied her somewhat. There was a large membrane covering the whole of one tonsil and extending over part of the soft palate. This was at 9.30 a.m. The case was forthwith removed to hospital. By 11 o'clock she was washed, warmed, and in bed, enjoying the comfort of hot bottles and the soothing influence of a steam-kettle and tent. By this time her pulse had somewhat improved, the croupy symptoms were lessened, and the medical attendant, who wished to see the injection of antitoxic serum, declared her condition somewhat improved. The membrane on the throat was one of the worst I have seen, coming away in large pieces and renewing very rapidly.

The next step was to verify the diagnosis, of which, however, there was no real doubt. Accordingly, I did not delay treatment. But a piece of membrane was detached, with the usual precautions, and put in a test-tube for examination by a bacteriologist.

Then, with every care against accidental

contamination, a dose of antitoxin was administered. Next day the membrane was not visibly altered. A second dose was given. On the third day the membrane was more easily detached. All croupy symptoms had gone. A third dose was given. The membrane completely disappeared. By the fourth day of treatment the throat was free of any sign of the disease. Local treatment was continued until there were no diphtheria bacilli left. The patient was, in due course, discharged. She showed no signs of paralysis.

Meanwhile, the hygienic forces had not been idle. The house, bed, bedclothes, bodyclothes, and other articles exposed to the infection had all been disinfected in the usual way.

This case shows how the public health organisation combines the various sciences to extirpate the disease and to preserve life. I shall now present, in more detail, the rational basis of the procedure.

That the Klebs-Löffler bacillus—a minute, rod-shaped organism—is a factor in diphtheria no one seriously disputes ; whether it is the whole cause, whether the chemical condition of the tissues is equally important, what precise part the glandular tissues of the throat play, and many other problems, are still matters open to argument. The Klebs-Löffler bacillus is at least a good diagnostic sign ; in doubtful cases it is the only early definite sign, and any physician who finds the micro-organism in a suspicious sore-throat is incurring a very grave responsibility if he fails to use the recognised methods of destroying it and its poisonous products. In matters of doubtful theory, it is well to give one's patient—not one's own prejudice—the benefit of the doubt

This micro-organism can be isolated from the diphtheritic membrane ; it grows readily in blood serum, or other suitable medium, at 95° Fahr. to 98·6° Fahr.,—that is, at about the temperature of the body,—and with the products of its activity diphtheria can be produced. In milk at this temperature the bacillus grows luxuriantly. "The diphtheria bacilli," says Klein, "are killed by heating to 60° Centigrade (*i.e.* 140° Fahr.) for five minutes." This bacillus affects rabbits, pigeons, cats, dogs, horses, calves, and milk cows. In the last—Klein holds it as proven—a form of pure cow diphtheria can be produced, and frequently is produced ; the eruption so caused on the teats may infect the milk, and thus may arise an epidemic of true human diphtheria. When the micro-organism alights on the human throat in an inflamed, or irritated, or raw, or ill-guarded condition, human diphtheria is the result.

Dr. Sidney Martin has determined the nature of the diphtheria poisons. The bacillus of diphtheria produces two orders of poisons—one found in the throat membrane, the other in the tissues, blood, and spleen of patients dead of diphtheria. The poison of the membrane acts probably as a ferment; at least, a single dose produces progressive paralysis, wasting, diarrhœa, and death. Examination after death shows nerve-degeneration, fatty degeneration of the skeletal muscles, and fatty degeneration of the heart. These results Dr. Martin has proved on warm-blooded animals such as rabbits. The other poisons—those found in the tissues—are similar to the substances produced by digestion in the stomach and small intestine. Being peculiar derivatives of albumen, these poisons are named " albumoses "—a class of physiological substances whose nature has been studied only within the last twenty-five years or so. The albumoses of diphtheria cause a rise of temperature (fever), increasing paralysis, difficulty of breathing, wasting, diarrhœa, nerve-degenerations, fatty degeneration of the heart, and fluidity of the blood after death. Some of these results follow the injection of other than diphtheritic albumoses. The ferment present in the membrane, on entering the body, acts on certain substances, and converts them into the albumoses mentioned. All the poisons are, therefore, directly or indirectly the result of the bacillus acting on special substances. The third poison—organic acid—produces certain nerve - degenerations, but not progressive paralysis.

Now, by the cultivation of the bacillus in appropriate media, all these poisons can be produced outside the body altogether ; they can be injected into the veins or tissues, and the results produced are the same as in true diphtheria. With these results before him, Dr. Martin concludes : " For these reasons, therefore, the bacillus diphtheriæ is the cause of diphtheria. . . . When the membrane is formed, the bacilli grow in it, especially near the surface, secrete a ferment which, when absorbed into the body, produces, by acting on the proteids of the body, digestive products, the chief of which belong to the albumose class. It is not that the body is poisoned by a single large dose, and then the action stopped (although this may occur in certain cases), but it is that numerous small doses are, in the course of the disease, absorbed into the system, and are gradually producing their effects." The action of these poisons, or toxins, it is that the antitoxin has to counteract. Dr. Martin's experiments on its power of counteraction are, so far as they go, equally decisive. His general conclusion is : " These experiments . . . tend to show that the antitoxic serum is capable of counteracting the poisons which are found in the tissues of patients dead of diphtheria. It has only a slight effect on the febrile rise of temperature produced by the albumose, but it completely counteracts the fatty degeneration of the heart produced by those substances, and to a great extent also the nerve-degeneration." Fifteen years of research have confirmed and extended these conclusions.

The case I have already described shows what part falls to the practical physician. The treatment of diphtheria all over the world is now based on the biological, chemical, and pathological results I have summarised. The physician's aim is twofold—first, to destroy the bacillus in the throat, and so to arrest the formation of the three orders of poisons ; second, to counteract the effects of the poisons (or toxins) already absorbed. The longer the disease has been allowed to go on the less chance there is of a cure, because the poisons act rapidly and may produce organic changes that are beyond cure.

For local treatment—that is, the destruction of the bacillus—a whole multitude of germicides have been recommended; cures have been claimed for them all, doubtless with more or less justice; but there is hardly one that, in other hands, has not resulted in keen disappointment. Much depends on the competence of the nurse. One solution was devised by Löffler himself. He experimented until he discovered a combination of drugs that could, without injuring the mucous membranes of the throat, destroy the Löffler bacillus in five seconds. Many reliable drugs could destroy it in twenty seconds or more. But this length of time made a proper application to the throat difficult. Löffler's solution has been in common use for many years. Löffler himself, when he introduced it, recorded that in ninety-six cases so treated there was not a single death. This is a good record, and he refers to cases in the early stage and markedly local. But even in these, one may fail from incompetent handling. But all such local treatment is immeasurably more satisfactory than sixteen years ago; for the patient is first made safe with anti-

toxin, and local treatment is no longer needed
for cure, but simply for the preventing of
fresh infection.

In the sixteen years that have passed since
this case occurred, the use of antitoxic serum
has spread all over the world. Cases in
hundreds of thousands have been treated.
The technique of dosage and injection have
been improved. Thus in a severe and late
case one very large dose is usually better than
several small doses. The serum is also
coming more and more into use as an immunising agent in advance. The death-rate from
diphtheria has continued to fall. Diphtheria
has lost much of its terror and all its hope-
lessness. To take but a single figure from
the Statistical Reports of the Metropolitan
Asylums Board. In 1894, the non-antitoxin days, of all the cases brought to all the
hospitals for treatment on the first day of the
disease, 22·5 per cent. died (133 cases, with
80 deaths). In the years 1895–96, the days
of antitoxin, of all the cases brought on the
first day for treatment, 8·8 per cent. died
(209 cases, with 8 deaths). The difference
between the methods when treatment is
delayed is less striking, but it is well on the
side of antitoxin. For instance, of 589 cases
treated on the second day, 27 per cent. died
under non-antitoxin treatment ; of 1126

cases, under antitoxin treatment, 12 per cent. died. In Chicago, in 1895, antitoxin began to be freely administered to the poor in their homes. The death-rate fell from 35 per cent. to 6 per cent. And the low death-rate has been on the whole maintained. Both in England and in Scotland, the Local Authorities for public health, with the consent and active approval of the Local Government Boards, have power to provide antitoxin free to every person suffering from the infection or requiring a protective dose.

The antitoxin of diphtheria has thus stood the most rigid tests both of laboratory experiment and of practical use. It has done more. It has led to the production of other antitoxins, whose use is only less known because, in this country, the diseases are less common.

Environmental factors always play a part in outbreaks of infection. In diphtheria, personal infection is, no doubt, the chief cause of spread. The bacillus is easily conveyed from the patient to any persons in his immediate neighbourhood. Indeed, it is probable that the chief reason why the number of cases occurring still remains so high is that " contacts " are not yet as thoroughly examined as in the great infections like smallpox and typhus. As the medical inspection of school children comes to closer grips with personal infection, the contacts of diphtheria will be as radically examined as those of smallpox, and diphtheria will receive another check.

But there are other factors, not least the type of season. It has been shown by Dr. Newsholme that " an epidemic of diphtheria never originates when there has been a series of years in which each year's rainfall is above the average amount. An epidemic of diphtheria never originates or continues in a wet year ... unless this wet year follows on two or more dry years immediately preceding it. The epidemics of diphtheria for which accurate data are available, have all originated in dry years."

The practical deduction from these conclusions is that diphtheria spreads more easily and more harmlessly in dry years, possibly because the conditions of the throats are then less fitted to give it a start within the body. Let the wet and cold season come, or let local conditions favour the occurrence of sore-throats and then we have a widespread and apparently sudden epidemic. The bacilli are lying on hundreds of tonsils, ready to grow dangerous when the throat inflames.

CHAPTER VI

HOW ANTITOXINS ARE PRODUCED AND PREPARED

FIFTEEN years ago circumstances found me in London.

" Have you been to The Poplars ? " inquired a medical friend.

" No," I answered. " Where is The Poplars ? "

" The Poplars," he said, " is the name of the farm at Sudbury in Middlesex where the anti-diphtheritic serum is prepared for the Lister Institute. Dr. Blank, from India, and I intend to drive out there to-morrow. Will you come ? "

" I should, with pleasure," I said, " but I fear my duties will prevent me."

And they did.

But on another day I took the train at Euston Station. Sudbury lies in Middlesex, to the north-west of London. From Euston it is only some eight miles by rail. The train sweeps you rapidly out of the new-laid north of London into a purely agricultural landscape. You pass Willesden, Harrow-on-the-Hill, and Wembley, until you come to a little country station that seems as far from London as the Glenkens of Galloway.

When I arrived at Sudbury I asked my way to The Poplars. The Poplars ? The first person was not certain ; he bade me inquire of a carrier, whose horse stood at a public-house door. Of him, then, I inquired ; but his knowledge was vague. " I think, sir, it is about a mile farther on, to the left-hand side." I walked onwards, over a dusty road, among rows of tall trees, and I was saluted everywhere with the charming and inimitable greenery of southern English landscapes. At last, guided by the map as much as by personal inquiry, I came to a farm—a dairy farm. " No, sir ; The Poplars is farther on." Every one that answered spoke of The Poplars in the most common tone of voice, as if one dairy farm were like another, and one green field not more than another green field. They showed no sign that within stone-throw of their door a miracle was going forward. The resources of science and the resources of nature were here coming to deadly grips, and the victory was less likely to be with nature than with science. Here the intellect of an inventive century was busy among the warp and woof of life, if haply one patch or pattern might yield up its secret. The tall trees near me, the green grass farther away; the farmyard living things here, the silent farmer there; the silent, still life made more silent and more still by the oppressive contrast with the tangled noises of London,—all came together in my imagination as I approached this farm of mystery, where the man of science, the Faust of our era, was busy with his alembics and his books of magic and wealth of learning that should save man from his sorrow. And I was reminded of the Spirit's reply to Faust when he was beginning to handle the instruments of mystery:

"In the currents of Life, in action's storm,
 I wander and I wave;
 Everywhere I be,
 Birth and the grave,
 An infinite sea,
 A web ever growing,
 A life ever flowing:
 Thus I weave at the loom of the years
 The garment of life that the Godhead wears."

At last I came on some roadside houses, which the Time Spirit seemed to treat kindly. *There* was The Poplars. I rang, and was admitted. In the room I recognised books and photographs and interests that belonged to my friend when we were at college together; and when the first doctor appeared I found him the same clear-eyed scientific idealist that I have known and admired for so many years—a gentleman from South Carolina, who came to learn the science of medicine at a Scottish University, and who now, after years of practical study, was still filling his mind with more mysteries of bacteriology. The doctor-in-chief — the director of this farm—came in about half an hour afterwards. He also was a fellow-graduate, and a contemporary of my own. It did not lessen the feeling of romance that two of the same University should have come—one from the North of Scotland, the other from the Southern States—to work out together and help to make the life-saving fluids that then raised our hopes so high. And more than ever I felt that here is your true man of practice : he labours night and day in the light of the pure intellect, adding fact to theory and developing theory from fact ; heeding neither day nor night, neither wealth nor poverty, neither comfort nor pain ; caring only for the truth and the good it may do. So long as life can offer us those free minds, ready to give themselves up to truth and the service of man, the world is going forward.

The afternoon was a lucky one. A telegram had been received the night before from Egypt for a supply of serum. Immediately on receipt of the telegram, the horse was bled and the blood subjected to all the operations necessary to separate off the serum and maintain it pure. These operations are very simple, and they apply to all the serums prepared—to the anti-diphtheritic serum among the rest. The horse is bled from the neck in the way familiar to the veterinary surgeon. The blood is received into a large flask, perfectly sterilised. In this flask it is allowed to sit until the clot separates from the serum. The serum is then decanted off and filtered through a Chamberland-Pasteur or a Berkefeld filter, under pressure of a small air-pump. This process is very slow ; the serum is more or less viscid, and, unlike water, it filters very slowly through the minute pores of the clay or porcelain. At every stage every precaution is taken against contamination, and the purpose of the filtration is to free the serum of any chance micro-organisms caught in the passage from the horse to the flask.

The next stage is the bottling, and it was my privilege to see the bottling of the first anti-choleraic serum ever drawn from a horse in Britain, possibly in the world. The process is very rapid and very precise. The two doctors and the laboratory boy take up

their places at a bench, the American on
the left, the director in the middle, the
laboratory boy on the right. Ready to the
hand of the American is a heap of small phials,
perfectly sterilised, and plugged with cotton-
wool. In front of him is the flask of filtered
serum. The flask has a hooded pipette.
Attached to this flask is a blow-pipe bellows
which he works by foot, so forcing the serum
through the pipette. To his right is a bunsen
burner. In front of the director lies a vessel
with indiarubber corks, also sterilised. In
front of the laboratory boy is a vessel of
melted paraffin, kept at boiling point. At a
signal from the director the work begins.
The American snatches a phial; with a
forceps, which he passes through the bunsen
flame, he removes over the flame the plug
of cotton-wool, instantly places the phial
under the hooded pipette, forces into it the
proper amount of serum, and hands it to the
director. He in turn has already taken up
a sterilised cork with a sterilised forceps;
instantly he fits the cork into the phial over
the flame, and hands the corked phial to
the laboratory boy. He in turn dips the
corked end into the boiling paraffin and
sets the phial down. These operations are
carried out so rapidly that some 600 phials
may be filled in an hour.

After the bottling, the phials are kept in an incubator for twenty-four hours, and, if possible, longer. If, at the end of the time, any one of a set shows the slightest sign of impurity or microbic life, the whole set is destroyed. Such is the care taken in the preparation of these delicate antidotes to those delicate and remorseless poisons.

Afterwards, I was taken round the farm, which had twenty-two horses, many rabbits, and guinea-pigs by the score. Among the horses the director pointed out the first pony that had ever yielded anti-diphtheritic serum in Britain. He had now ceased to yield any ; but he was kept as an interesting old friend, and he was quietly enjoying the life he had so well earned by his blood.

Diphtheria has here a perfectly definite meaning ; it yields its poison ; it produces its definite sequences of morbid phenomena ; it produces its antidote. At every stage it is under control ; its actions and reactions can be predicted ; its precise strength can be measured ; it can be neutralised to a perfect nicety. I was shown about a pint and a half of diphtheria fluid, which, so I was informed, was the most concentrated and strongest diphtheria poison hitherto produced in the world. Yet it was in use there to produce definite, predictable results.

How is antitoxin produced ? It is produced by slowly immunising a horse against diphtheria. The process of immunisation takes five or six months to accomplish. The dose of diphtheria toxin is increased slowly, but never so as to put the animal in danger. At a certain stage the blood and tissues acquire complete immunity to diphtheria, and the largest dose of virulent diphtheria that can be conveniently injected into the blood will fail to produce the slightest evidence of disease. It is then that the horse's blood-serum is ready to be used as an antitoxin. The process of preparing it, I have already described.

If the same course of graduated doses of toxin could be carried out in the human being, the same process of immunisation would result Indeed, such a process of partial immunisation probably does result in " carrier cases " of diphtheria. Diphtheria, it has been conclusively shown, spreads from person to person in the dry seasons ; it grows mildly in the throat without producing symptoms, and in the course of its growth probably confers a certain immunity. Unfortunately, it is not practically possible so to inoculate the throat as to graduate the doses and the partial immunity otherwise occurring cannot be relied upon. When the child has only hours to live, he must have the benefit of the most rapid remedy, which is the flooding of the body with an antidote.

Antitoxins of some other diseases have been prepared in a similar way. Thus a horse can be immunised against lockjaw, and the resulting antitoxin, though it has not had the striking success of diphtheria antitoxin, has shown great curative power. Lockjaw (tetanus) is probably the most deadly of diseases, and it is usually well established before antitoxin can be applied. An antitoxin, too, has been prepared from cholera ; but hitherto its success as a cure has not been established.

The immunity produced by antitoxin is not permanent. In diphtheria, it passes away in a few months. A person may have a second and a third and a fourth attack. Further, the antitoxin does not itself kill the bacillus of diphtheria. It is not a microbicide. To inject antitoxin, therefore, is never by itself an adequate treatment of diphtheria ; the throat and nose must also be sterilised ; for, although the patient himself is made immune, the bacilli can grow on his tissues and retain all their former virulence.

CHAPTER VII

IMMUNITY—NATURAL AND ACQUIRED

A DIRTY pin-prick may produce an inflammation of the finger. What is inflammation ? Its cardinal marks, recorded from the most ancient days of surgery, are—redness, swelling, heat, pain. The pain comes from the irritation of the nerve-endings. The heat comes from the increased circulation of hot blood at the surface. The swelling comes from the distention of the blood-vessels, the concentration of blood-cells and exudation of fluid from the vessels. The redness also comes from the local increase of the blood supply. These are familiar facts ; but they contain some of the most difficult problems in the biology of disease.

Assume that the dirt on the pin-point has been a minute round germ,—a micrococcus. Assume, too, that on the given pin-point there were some thousands of micrococci. Their minute size allows us to make the assumption. For the moment, neglect the mechanical effect of the pin itself. Let us attend only to the micrococcus. The moment it is through the skin, it begins its work. Its numbers are soon doubled and quadrupled, and rapidly become millions. To this the blood and blood-vessels reply by a series of changes. The minute arteries dilate ; the minute veins dilate ; the blood-stream is quickened. After a time, the blood-stream slows down, and the white blood-cells, separating from the red, glide along the walls of the most minute vessels. At last the stream stops ; the minute vessels are filled with red and white blood-cells— the white adhering in many places to the side of the vessels. Then there is an exudation of fluid through the vessels into the tissue. Following this, white blood-cells squeeze through the vessel-walls and, in their thousands and millions, gather round the point of disturbance.

Then the battle between the white cells and the micrococci begins. Rapidly the jelly-like cell alters its shape, steadily surrounds one microbe after another, until its body contains ten, fifty, one hundred or more. If the conditions are favourable to the white cells, the battle goes on until every microbe is absorbed by a cell, until the exudation, solid or liquid, is all reabsorbed, and until the circulation of the blood in the part again becomes normal.

But, if the conditions are favourable to the micrococci, the issue is very different.

Their numbers may be too great; then millions of white cells die in the struggle, their bodies perhaps breaking up and liberating small quantities of antitoxin. The micrococci, too, die in their millions; but their rate of increase is enormous, and they continue to advance. To meet them come millions more of the white cells, absorbing their enemies, digesting them, and producing the antidote to the microbic poison. If, at last, the white cell conquers, the process of repair goes on as before; but now the process takes longer, for an abscess, containing the dead white cells, has been formed, and some of the fixed tissues have been destroyed. If the white cells on the outskirts of the abscess could be examined, they would be found gorged with micrococci. The rapid mobilisation of the white cells in response to the violent stimulus has been enough to stop the invasion.

If, however, the conditions continue to be less favourable to the white cells, and more favourable to the micrococci, the cells may be killed in millions more, their cordon may be broken through, and the microbes may pass into the larger vessels of the body, so causing a general infection. Even then, the work of the white cells continues; in the blood, it may meet the microbe and absorb it as before. In the glands, it does the same; everywhere, it goes on devouring the microbes and producing its antitoxin, until, at last, the microbe meets its antidote everywhere, and its warfare fails. If, however, the conditions are still unfavourable to the white cells, the microbe, dying in millions, produces more millions to continue the invasion. The war goes on until every defence is broken down; then the slight inflammation of the pricked finger ends in a fatal blood-poisoning.

What are the conditions favourable to the white cells ? The conditions are many, but some are cardinal

The blood has in it some substances that make it easier for the white cell (or leucocyte) to take in the microbe. These substances are the opsonins—the discovery of Sir Almroth Wright. The name opsonin is formed from the Greek word *opson*, which means a sauce, or seasoning, anything that makes the morsel more tempting. If the blood is rich in opsonins, the leucocytes, when a germ whose opsonin is present enters, win the fight; for they find the germs, thus prepared, easy to absorb and digest. And the opsonins are, possibly, of as many kinds as the germs that enter. But here there is much dispute among experts. Probably there is a common opsonin, which may, in some degree, act as a sauce to every microbe; but there are certainly special opsonins, and on these depends the readiness of the special microbe to be eaten by the leucocyte. To the eating leucocyte let us also give its technical name—phagocyte (eating cell).

What are the special opsonins ? They are probably the opsonins produced by the action of the special microbe itself. They are regarded as substances distinct from toxins.

In diphtheria we saw that the toxin in the blood results in the production of an antitoxin. In many other cases, there is a parallel result. If the lockjaw (tetanus) toxin is introduced, the result is a specific antitoxin. If the tubercle bacillus is introduced, the result is an antidote to tubercle. If the typhoid bacillus is introduced, the result is an antidote to typhoid. The times and quantities vary, but the general reaction is the same. And it is not confined to microbes. If cells from a kidney are introduced into the blood, the result is an antitoxic substance that destroys the tube-lining of the normal kidney. If liver cells are introduced, there is a similar result for the cells of the liver. And there are many other substances that once introduced into the blood produce similar anti-substances. In every case, whether the agent be a microbe or other substance, the dose, if it is to produce the result, has to be carefully adjusted ; but the result always occurs. It is, then, possible to make a wide general proposition, —certain substances produce anti-substances. But the substances that produce these extraordinary effects have one thing in common : they all have a somewhat similar chemical composition.

To return now to the opsonins. Every infectious fever probably leaves behind more or less of its particular opsonin. When, therefore, the microbe of the fever re-enters the blood, it is more easily absorbed and digested by the phagocyte. It may re-enter a hundred times, but it never breaks down the first line of defence. So long as this condition remains, the patient is safe against a second attack. When the condition disappears, he may become as liable to an attack as ever. But one attack confers a passing or permanent immunity against another.

Let us add another technical point. Assume two persons—one a person in normal health, the other infected with the tubercle bacillus. Take from the body of each some of their leucocytes. Prepare, also, a culture of the tubercle bacillus, which can now, thanks to the methods made familiar by Koch in 1881, be easily cultivated. Let us now make two experiments. Mix the leucocytes of the normal person with a certain quantity of the tubercle bacilli. Mix the leucocytes of the tubercular person with a certain other quantity of the bacilli. Keep both the mixtures at the proper temperature for a quarter of an hour or so. Then make two microscopic preparations, one from the normal person's mixture, the other from the infected person's mixture. Examine each under the microscope and note the difference. Select, say, fifty leucocytes, and count the number of bacilli they have eaten in the time. The counting is difficult, but it can be done by a skilled eye. Add up the numbers found in each of the fifty cells, and divide the total by fifty. This gives the average for each cell. Do the same with the infected person's cells. Let us suppose that in each cell of the normal person we have found on the average 125 bacilli ; in each cell of the infected person we have found on the average 75. Make these two numbers into a fraction—75 as numerator, 125 as denominator—which is three-fifths, or in decimals 0·6. This is the " opsonic index."

Here I have omitted the delicate and complicated technique, which is one of the marvels of modern insight and invention. It is enough that we get a general understanding of the opsonic index. And it is important that the term opsonic index should become familiar to everybody ; for, like the term phagocyte, it is part of a system of marvellous discoveries, a world by itself, a kingdom where only the skilled have entry, and they only after years of laborious toil.

The opsonic index, then, is an index of relative powers of resistance. If, in our particular case, the resistance of the healthy person be counted as one, the resistance of the infected person would be only three-fifths. A healthy person's resistance to tubercle is, therefore, greater than the infected person's resistance. If, therefore, they were both equally exposed to a fresh dose of the tubercle infection, the healthy person would throw off the attack much more effectively than the person already infected. When the opsonic index is high, the leucocytes can absorb and destroy germs in much greater quantity than when the opsonic index is low. When, therefore, the index is high, the resistance is great ; when the index is low, the resistance is feeble.

If this be so, the question at once is suggested : Is it possible to heighten the opsonic index when it is low ? It is possible to answer " yes." And this answer has a claim to be called the greatest departure in modern medicine. Here, at last, it seems, prevention and cure pass into a perfect synthesis.

This is a broad outline of Metchnikoff's theory of phagocytosis—the theory that the white blood cells, by absorbing microbes and other foreign invaders, defend the body from infection and probably from some other poisons too. The theory is not universally accepted ; but it has a vast mass of experimental research to rest upon. The action of the white cell is not an isolated fact. It has many parallels among the lower animals. The white cell is itself a living organism. In the blood, it acts as if it were a free animal. It searches for food, it meets aggressors, it adapts itself to dangers, it is attracted by some chemical conditions, it is repelled by others. Some microbes, therefore, it will absorb and digest ; some it will permit to pass into the circulation. In the one case, it prevents infection ; in the other case, it permits infection. Why it takes to one and leaves the other, is not easy to explain. Possibly some microbes produce a substance that attracts a leucocyte ; some, a substance that repels. There are facts in favour of this idea. There are, however, cases that the phagocyte (eater-cell) theory does not directly cover. In diphtheria, the poisonous agent is not a microbe, but a soluble toxin. Does the antitoxin come from the phagocyte ? Possibly it does ; possibly the phagocyte secretes the antitoxin and sets it free in the blood.

These disputable details need not be pursued. The theory is fascinating, even romantic, but full of difficulties. Yet it correlates an immense range of facts in the animal world. It brings protection against infectious diseases into line with many other natural processes. It puts before us a protective material mechanism, visible, definite, capable of experimental test. And it is not incompatible with other theories of immunity.

For the present, no one theory holds the field. But the chief accepted fact is—that when microbes, blood-cells, tissue-cells, and other substances chemically allied to them, are injected into the blood, they stimulate the blood, its cells, and the cells of the fixed tissues to produce anti-substances, which are antidotes to the substances injected. Let this be granted. It in no way conflicts with the theory of phagocytosis. It is, too, enough for the ends of immediate practice ; because, relying on this general truth, we can prevent or stay the progress of certain diseases by injecting " vaccines " prepared from the microbes that produce the disease. The preparation of such vaccines is a highly technical process, but it is entirely practicable, and is now very widely practised. The essential principle of the method is that the microbe of the given disease is carefully cultivated, until it is a pure culture. It is then by sterilisation rendered incapable of reproducing itself in the blood, but it is not robbed of its power to produce immunity. There is in the substance of the microbe's own body a substance that induces the formation of an anti-substance. The aim of the treatment is to produce this anti-substance for the given disease. When the anti-substance is produced in the blood and tissues, the disease is cured and immunity against it is established.

Many diseases are treated on these lines. For instance, acne or " pimples," boils, common colds.

Of the greater diseases so treated, the greatest is tuberculosis. Early in his researches, Koch discovered that the tubercle bacilli contained a special substance in their bodies This he named tuberculin. It is now known as Koch's " old tuberculin," because of its method of preparation. It is used all over the world, mainly for the purposes of diagnosis. Wherever tuberculosis of any kind is present in a patient's body, tuberculin, injected in a minute and harmless dose, produces a slight fever. This reaction is a proof that tuberculosis is present.

Recently the method of applying tuberculin has been simplified. Calmette applied it to the conjunctiva, the external membrane of the eye. It produces there a local and evanescent inflammation, but only if the patient is tubercular. To von Pirquet we owe a further improvement. He applies it to the skin. This results in a definite local reaction, wherever there is or has been tubercular disease. It is, indeed, almost too delicate a test for practice. Among the inmates of one asylum in Scotland it indicated that some 70 per cent. of patients had all, at some time in their lives, suffered from tuberculosis. Dr. Herford, Altona, with the consent of the parents, applied the test to 2594 school children. Of these, 63 per cent. reacted. Of the five-year-old groups, 50 per cent. reacted. Of those about to leave school, that is, the thirteen- and fourteen-year-old groups, 94 per cent. reacted.

These facts are confirmed by other researches. They prove the extreme delicacy of the test and the practical universality of some degree of tuberculosis.

For treatment, too, tuberculin has been used in several forms. One of the commonest forms is Koch's TR or new tuberculin. Some form of tuberculin has been in more or less constant use for treatment ever since Koch first discovered it. But recently the " old tuberculin " has been confined to diagnosis. The " new tuberculin " and preparations based on it are alone used for treatment.

Sir Almroth Wright, in working out his opsonic index theory, found that, when a small quantity of tuberculin is injected into a tubercular patient, the first and immediate result is that the capacity of the phagocytes goes down. There is a " negative phase." The susceptibility to the spread of the infection within the body is, for the time, increased. In a few days, the negative phase passes away and, in the end, the opsonic index reaches a higher level than before the injection. The capacity of the phagocytes is increased. Thus, by watching the rise and fall of the opsonic index, the physician can determine when it is most profitable to give a second and a third and a fourth injection.

This, incidentally, bears out what is said below of unborn children of tubercular fathers and mothers (p. 128). The disease will take no account of the " negative phase," though occasionally it may pass into the child when his negative phase is ending and then the infection will be curative. But, often as not, it will reduce the capacity of the embryonic phagocytes, so increasing the susceptibility of the child to tuberculosis. But this is all a matter of chance for the unborn child. It is a matter of precise science for the patient under treatment.

After long and laborious trials, the experts are now able to gauge the correct dose of tuberculin. It may be as small as the 10,000th part of a milligramme of the solid tuberculin, that is about the 650,000th part of a grain. The dose can be slowly increased, the opsonic index being taken from time to time, or some similar test being applied, to ensure that the patient's immunity is not being reduced instead of increased.

Now that the way is made clear, the use of tuberculin is increasing steadily everywhere for all forms of tuberculosis,—glands, bones, etc. In a short time the injection of tuberculin will be as familiar as vaccination for smallpox. The stupid haste of twenty years ago in working without first ascertaining the correct dose did harm, but the reaction due to it has now passed away. The secrets of the method are now revealing themselves outside the laboratories. The administrative bodies thus obtain a new instrument of immense value. If the hopes now stirred by tuberculin are even in small part realised, the drop in the death-rate from tuberculosis will soon astonish the world. The fight between the greater and the lesser organism, the human body and this remorseless parasite, will be changed into a friendly and continuous process of immunisation. And so the terrors of heredity will be once more put to confusion; for to be born of mildly tubercular stock may yet become the best certificate of physical and ethical fitness. The stone that the builders rejected may become the head of the corner.

CHAPTER VIII

A DISCUSSION OF THE TUBERCULAR DIATHESIS

It is now profitable to ask the question: Is immunity to a particular disease ever inherited ? Is a predisposition to a particular disease ever inherited ? What is meant by diathesis, or predisposition to a particular disease ?

These questions it is well to ask; for they are questions of the hour and affect fundamentally the practice of life. In particular, it is well to discuss the meaning of diathesis; for it is frequently flung at the administrator to prove the futility of his administration. If I had taken at face value half of what I had been taught about heredity and diathesis, I should probably not have thought it worth while to enter the public health service. Further, as the tubercular diathesis is at present the focus of violent disputes, I prefer to investigate its meaning before passing on to discuss the control of tuberculosis.

Opium produces sleep because it has a *virtus dormitiva*—a dormitive virtue. This is the classical gibe at the metaphysics of the Middle Ages — the metaphysics that Comte's Positivism is supposed to have superseded. But the dormitive-virtue theory of opium was at least in line with the science of its own day. It was as good as the concept of material substance to " explain " matter, or mental substance to " explain " mind. But somehow men are slow to give up this way of satisfying their intellectual desires. They love to repeat to themselves in their answer precisely what they put to themselves

in their question. Does not pharmacy with
its " essences " keep alive for us the names
of no end of mediaeval ghosts ? And can
we say that anywhere our language has
shaken itself free of them ? But I am not
now thinking of differentiations of language,
which, of course, do not always keep pace
with the realities of thought. If the doctor
accidentally uses ancient terms, he is not
often misled by them either in his diagnosis
or in his treatment. But there are some
terms that are still doing as much harm
to clear thinking as the worst that can be
selected from mediaeval medicine.

Take, for instance, the term " diathesis."
How often we heard the word when we were
students ! What a thrill of pleasure we had
when we were first able to write down of our
own motion that our patient was an illustration of the " Tubercular Diathesis " !
We looked for every feature—the transparent
skin, the long eyelash, the fragile frame ; or
again, the coarse skin, the thick lip, and all
the correlated items of the classical descriptions. It was with a sense of intellectual
finality that we heard scrofula defined as a
" vulnerability " of the tissues, particularly
of the skin and mucous membranes. The
words did more than satisfy our intellectual
emotions. They positively stopped the im-

pulse to question the teacher. They remained for years in our minds as a solvent of new difficulties, an obstruction to new mental growths, blessed words of perfected science. They were like Spencer's Evolution formula —a thing first to learn by heart and then to fit on to everything that happened, not minding much whether a finger of the glove was only half on, or, indeed, whether there was anything particular for the glove to fit on to.

Then there was our first case of rheumatism —the " rheumatic diathesis." We searched the text-books for the exact characterisation of this typical state of human flesh. It was not merely a disease we were contemplating ; it was a history, a whole theory of the organism, a metaphysic of all the symptoms.

Then there was the " gouty diathesis." How much it counted for ! Gout was the name for the possessing spirit, the demon that proceeded to the toe or retroceded to the stomach, producing wherever he went fresh evil and pain. Sometimes, perhaps, he was called " gout " because the patient could not spell " rheumatism." But gouty or rheumatic, it was always " diathesis," and there our minds rested, blocked with a beautiful Greek word, silenced by the genius of the Ægean Sea.

I have often wondered who introduced the term " diathesis." He is one of the benefactors of the race. His word is an indispensable term in the litany of the medical religion—the *Religio Medici*. What should we do without its emotional suggestion, its capacity for satisfying intellectual desire ? No plain Saxon word like " set " or " through-set " could give us the touch of mystery that " diathesis " gives. It will hold its ground in the litany for many generations ; because it comes trippingly on the tongue and not offends the ear. There is, of course, the word temperament—the melancholic, lymphatic, etc. But " temperament " is Latin, " diathesis " is Greek, and there is a subtle difference between them that only spiritual experience enables us to discern.

Shall we leave this beautiful word to continue its gentle ministrations to our intellectual life ? Or dare we ask whether the time has not come for testing its credentials ?

This question I should never have thought of asking but that recently I have had to read a good deal about tuberculosis. On every hand I have been silenced by the " tubercular diathesis." When I expressed the belief that the tubercle bacillus was the chief cause of tuberculosis, the body being for the time a medium of infinite complexity and offering a thousand varieties of food for the parasite, I was always met with—" Yes, but there is the diathesis. You must take that into account." And it was explained to me that there was something that made some people " predisposed " to phthisis and left others " unpredisposed." When I pressed to know what " predisposed " meant, I found it was another name for the " diathesis," and, indeed, it is pretty much the Latin of which diathesis is the Greek. Sometimes I had thrown at me the whole word " predisposition," as if, being longer, it might produce more psychological effect than " diathesis." And it did ; just because it was longer, but for no other reason. When I pressed the further question, what evidence there is of a tubercular diathesis or predisposition, I was answered: " The fact that the person takes tuberculosis." Thus my education was advancing ; for now I had got into a circle—a vicious circle. The tubercular diathesis makes it easy for a person to contract tuberculosis ; that he contracts tuberculosis proves that he has the tubercular diathesis. When I pointed this out to my tutor, he said: " Yes, yes, that may be logical ; but we are not dealing with logic, we are dealing with facts."

And then he proceeded to detail to me,

with instance upon instance, how the " fairy type " falls a victim to the bacillus in spite of every conceivable precaution ; how the coarse-skinned type equally falls a victim, and nothing will either prevent his fall or slow down the progress of the disease. He explained to me by what tests I should know the various types, and that I need never mistake them. These had survived in the course of selection as the " vulnerable " types, clothed with a skin of extreme vulnerability, the victim being non-resistant in tissue, keen in brain, precocious, restless, fragile, near to genius. I am not sure that he did not also tell me about Wright's discovery of the opsonic index, by which you can invariably tell the true " tubercular diathesis."

These " facts " were very persuasive. It did seem as if we could, after all, determine by objective marks whether a tubercular diathesis existed, and could from it predict the probability of subsequent infection. But I was still puzzled as to why, in the course of racial evolution, such types should have survived at all. It is a truism that all men are different, some being born with one susceptibility in the ascendant, others with another ; some to honour, some to dishonour. This I could accept. The man of six feet will usually have a longer stroke at golf than a man of four feet, and if the race of life were a game of golf we could predict that the longer arm would have the shorter score. But the " tubercular diathesis " seemed to me a little more complicated. It is so Protean in its embodiments. At one time it is clothed in fat ; at another time it is thin and pale. At one time it is coarse, sallow, dark-haired, thick-lipped ; at another time it is fine, pink-skinned, blue-veined, long-eyelashed, fair-haired, with a delicate woolly hair on the body. Its forms have a variety suspiciously resembling the forms of real tuberculosis. And as I thought of this, the suspicion flashed upon me—" Can the diathesis after all be an undiagnosed case of real tuberculosis ? Is the thick-lipped, scrofulous child not already suffering from the actual infection of tuberculosis ? Is the fair-haired, thin-skinned, pink-cheeked fairy not already also suffering from the toxic effects of the bacillus ? "

Then, looking backward, I remembered just such a beautiful fairy, nine years old. She came of a highly tubercular family, father and mother being alike affected. One day swellings came on in the cheeks, and the doctor diagnosed mumps, which was then going the round. But ultimately he

found that the swellings were due to diphtheria. She then came into my hands;
but too late for antitoxin to save her. She
died of cardiac collapse at the end of three
days. All her tissues were eminently
" vulnerable." The needle of the syringe
caused a considerable hæmorrhage under
the skin. Her " tissue-resonance," as it
were, was very high. After she died I
found diseased glands in the chest and in
the abdomen; some of them were well on
the way to considerable abscesses. Yet the
child had been at school until the day her
cheeks began to swell, and had shown practically no symptom of serious ill-health. She
had always been " delicate." One would
have called her a typical instance of the
" fairy type " of the tubercular " diathesis."
She was, in fact, a perfect type of actual
tuberculosis.

Then I began to look for our positive
evidence of the existence of a special tubercular diathesis. Have we, after all, been
accepting this term too uncritically ? What
tests have we applied to the " fairy " or the
" coarse " types of the diathesis ? Have
we done anything whatever to show that,
by the time they exhibit signs of the diathesis,
they have not already been for months or

years infected with tuberculosis ? In fact, I now put the question—May not the so-called diathesis be itself the product of the tubercle bacillus ? Do we not simply assume that the diathesis is a fact without making any effort to prove that it is a fiction ?

Consider the chances that the child of one year has of acquiring tuberculosis. At birth, it is impossible to say by simple observation whether the child illustrates the tubercular diathesis or not. He must be at least several months, more probably years, old before we can say with certainty, There is the " fairy type." He must have the thick scrofulous lip before we can say, There is the " scrofulous type." But the infant has to be fed at least six or eight times a day for a year. Roughly, he will receive three thousand diets in his first year. That is, he may have three thousand prolonged opportunities of swallowing tubercle germs. And he has fifty thousand shorter opportunities of absorbing them from his fingers, from the floor, from clothing, from sucking-bottles, from his mother's fingers, and from all the other paraphernalia that constitute the environment of the infant. With this enormous potentiality of infection, who shall say that, by the time he exhibits the signs of the " fairy type," he is not already well advanced in tuberculosis ?

The signs of the so-called tubercular diathesis, therefore, may be themselves signs of infantile tuberculosis, and as yet we have no proof that they are not. If it should turn out that the " fairy types " are really tubercular patients, we shall have helped to exorcise one more ghost from our heritage of mediaevalism.

If there is a tubercular diathesis, there must also be the following : the smallpox diathesis, the cow-pox diathesis, the chicken-pox diathesis, the measles diathesis, the scarlet fever diathesis, the typhus diathesis, the typhoid diathesis, the plague diathesis, the diphtheria diathesis, the cerebro-spinal fever diathesis, the cholera diathesis, the whooping-cough diathesis, the influenza diathesis, the mumps diathesis, the erysipelas diathesis, the septicæmia diathesis, the tetanus diathesis, and as many more as there are specific infectious diseases now known or yet to be discovered. We might go even further. We might add a diathesis for each peculiarity that adapts the human body as a soil for any special germ or any parasite, whether it produces disease or not. For instance, there would be the ringworm diathesis, the favus diathesis, the scabies diathesis, and so on.

If we understand clearly that the term

diathesis means only the fact that the human body is adapted to the growth of the micro-organism, if it is only a short way of saying that the micro-organism can grow in the body, no one can object to that use of the word. But for the term tubercular diathesis there is a further claim made. It is maintained that we have definite signs of its existence before the individual under examination actually contracts the infection or could have been subject to tubercular toxins. This is a very large assumption when we reflect that any person might be exposed to tubercular toxins even before birth.

Doubtless, if we had methods of the requisite delicacy, we could, in every instance, find out precisely what conditions of the body make it possible for each individual germ to grow. We should know why the human being takes smallpox, and diathesis would be a name for our discovery. But, for the present, to call it so adds nothing to our knowledge, and does not help us in the least to understand the conditions. The word serves only as a convenient label of an unexplained fact. The same would be true of scarlet fever diathesis and all the others. But once the term diathesis is thus reduced to its legitimate meaning, as simply a name for the fact that if you take scarlet fever, you must first have been capable of taking it, all the emotional value evaporates, and we turn to other gods. The term is then an " honest ghost," but it unravels no mysteries. Is it not time that medicine gave up the *virtus dormitiva* method of describing its problems ? Would it not better serve the ends of science if the terminology were kept scientific ? Why load the student's mind with those myths, those superstitions of the pre-scientific days ? Or, to put it lower down still, why cannot we describe our qualities by adjectives, and not by abstract nouns, which always tend to " go off on their own," and afterwards return to dominate our intelligence instead of serving it ?

That the question is not unimportant practically is proved by the recent discussion at the International Anti-Tuberculosis Association. Experts from every country took part in the discussion. The old view has its adherents ; but the new view seems to gain ground. That some people take tuberculosis more easily than others goes without saying. They are, it may be, born with the disposition. That is not the question in dispute. The question is,—how is the disposition produced ? Is it an inherited variation of the germ-plasm, or a condition acquired by the child before birth, because the father, or mother, or both, are themselves infected and have communicated to their child the microbe or some of its toxins ?

On the answer to the question largely depends the method of prevention. If the condition commonly described as tubercular diathesis be itself a condition of actual tuberculosis, it offers no explanation of predisposition. Do the human tissues have any property that enables the tubercle bacillus to grow on them ? Undoubtedly. It is this property that has to be accounted for. Does the property vary in different individuals ? Most probably it does. Lines of possible explanation are indicated in the theory of phagocytosis and other theories of natural or acquired immunity. The phagocytes have a general capacity for capturing and destroying all intruding microbes. This would be, for the human being, a *general* " diathesis " against infectious diseases. The phagocytes may also have a special capacity for capturing and destroying particular microbes, like the tubercle bacillus. This, if inherited, would be a *special* " diathesis " against tubercle. This special capacity may depend on the presence of certain opsonins or other conditions.   The point in dispute is this : Is this special capacity for capturing and destroying the tubercle bacillus genuinely inherited as a physical peculiarity of healthy stock, or is it acquired by the individual either through infection from the parents or from some other outside source ?

It is admitted that the advance of tuberculosis in the body depends on the dose of tubercle administered.   If the dose is large, the advance is rapid.   If the dose is carefully graduated, not only does the disease not advance, it slows down and stops.   And it is possible to inoculate any healthy person with tubercle bacilli.   It is probable that any person whatsoever may be so reduced in resistance to disease in general, or so grossly dosed with virulent preparations of the tubercle bacillus, that he will develop the disease in its full strength.   The predisposition, or special capacity, can, therefore, be produced if the trouble is taken to produce it. Measles probably increases the predisposition or susceptibility of children to tuberculosis.

The mere fact, therefore, that children born of tubercular fathers and mothers do, in exceptional numbers, contract tuberculosis, does not prove that, in the healthy state, their tissues are exceptionally susceptible ; for there is, by hypothesis, no obtainable evidence that their tissues were ever in a healthy state. Before conception they may have been poisoned on the father's side or on the mother's side, as is known to occur in syphilis ; after conception they may have been continually poisoned during the whole period from conception to birth. If, after birth, they show signs of exceptional predisposition, this is precisely what, by hypothesis, we should expect. If any human body has been subjected to persistent doses of a poison, we are entitled to look for either of two results—greater susceptibility to the poison or partial immunisation. It is possible that those born with the so-called tubercular diathesis are those in whom the ante-natal doses have broken down the natural resistance, and that those born without the so-called diathesis are those in whom the doses have been such as to produce partial immunity.

The infinite variety of the disease in fathers and mothers makes these suppositions perfectly legitimate. We know that, in tuberculosis, it is possible, by careful graduation of the dose of tuberculin, to confer immunity on the patient ; but the graduation of the dose is difficult, and, in unskilled hands, the immunity might be lessened instead of increased. It may be so in the unborn infant,—sometimes its resistance (natural immunity) may be lessened, sometimes increased. If it be possible, in perfectly healthy tissue, to increase the susceptibility to tuberculosis —and there is much evidence to show that this is possible—there is no need to assume any special variation of the human germ-plasm. Any germ-plasm exposed to the disease in the father's or mother's body may have its natural capacity to grow the bacillus increased. The original natural capacity to grow the bacillus, like the capacity to grow the bacillus of smallpox, or typhoid, or scarlet fever, is legitimately named "diathesis." But the special predisposition produced by the paternal or maternal infection or poisoning is not in the strict sense a " diathesis," a fundamental quality of the healthy tissue that will develop whether the body is ever exposed to the infection or not. Such a special predisposition is not " inherited." It is an " acquired character." It is made up of two elements—an original capacity to grow the bacillus on the tissue, and a specially developed capacity induced by the actual presence of the bacillus or its poisons, a prolonged and predominant " negative phase." The original capacity to grow the bacillus is, of course, inherited like any other physical peculiarity. That is only another way of saying that we can take the disease. But, if the bacillus were a flea or a bug, we should not think of inventing a flea-diathesis or a bug-diathesis to account for the fact that the insects can live on our body juices. But if an attack of bugs could increase our body's attraction for bugs, we should then possess both an original capacity for feeding bugs and a special predisposition (acquired) for being fed on by them.

In the discussion of immunity we saw that the conditions of natural, or apparently natural, immunity alter by very fine shades. If Metchnikoff's view that animals are immune to cholera because their intestines contain a special microbe that kills the microbe of cholera be correct, the immunity of animals to cholera is not, in our sense, a diathesis ; it is possibly an accident of the food environment. Change the food, and the animal's immunity may disappear. Or change the food of the human being, and he may become immune. The extraordinary facts revealed by the " soured milk " treatment—treatment with lactic-acid-producing bacilli—make such a suggestion reasonable. Probably many of the states we are all too ready to regard as inherited are after all only acquired characters subtly masked.

The more the causes of immunity are found to belong to the environment, the more manageable will they become, and we shall not always be met with the insuperability of the "intensity of inheritance." That the environment counts even in the very stable immunities is certain. It is known that disturbances of digestion may predispose to cholera. Immunity, says Dr. Tanner Hewlett, is perhaps never absolute. It may alter with trifling alterations in the chemical composition of the blood. It may disappear when there is a change in the animal's temperature or in the external temperature. It may be complete for a specific germ acting alone, but incomplete for the same germ acting with another. It may rise or fall with fatigue. And there are many other special conditions that cause it to vary.

To take another illustration,—no one suggests that, when a child is born with syphilis, the reason is because it inherited from its syphilitic parent or parents the " syphilitic diathesis." It is known that the child shows symptoms of syphilis because it has contracted syphilis directly from the father or mother. It is also known that "the syphilitic diathesis," the capacity to contract the infection of syphilis, is universal among mankind. It is not so among the animals ; only a few of the higher animals are capable of contracting the infection. They have not the " syphilitic diathesis." On the contrary, they have " the anti-syphilitic diathesis." Not to load a discussion with needless refinements, let it, then, be said that if " tubercular diathesis " is to run on all-fours with the syphilitic diathesis, if it is to be regarded as universal among mankind, no one need object to the term ; but the inferences based on the hypothesis that it is not universal among mankind fall to the ground.

But a more serious point remains. The tuberculin test as now applied on the skin (von Pirquet's test) indicates that probably fifty, sixty, seventy, or even ninety per cent. of the general population suffer or have, at some period of their lives, suffered from some degree of tuberculosis. It is also known that tuberculosis contracted in infancy may lie latent for many years. It is also reasonably conjectured that, in later life, the apparent infection from an outside source is not really a new infection, but a flaming-up of the old infection into activity. If these facts be so, and the evidence in their favour steadily accumulates, our conclusions on " the intensity of inheritance " need re-interpretation. How much of apparent tuberculosis is due to a truly inherited variation, how much to conditions of evil nurture, how much to the assaults of other diseases, how much to accidental intoxications by other organisms, how much to the absence of protecting organisms in the bowel, how much to wrong habits of food,—these and many other problems must then be subjected to a new analysis.

Meanwhile, as administrative activity increases, the death-rate from tuberculosis diminishes ; but the few thousands of lives that will be saved in the years coming need not terrify the Eugenists or seriously hamper the man of science in his search for a more complete theory. The King's government *must* be carried on !

CHAPTER IX

THE ADMINISTRATIVE ASPECTS OF TUBERCULOSIS

How does the problem of tuberculosis present itself to the administrative mind ? To that question I shall try to give some answer.

For the modern administrator, the history

of tuberculosis began when Koch isolated
his bacillus. That the disease was an infection, communicable from man to man, is
a fact as old at least as the days of Isocrates,
and older. Through the ages, the belief
in its infectivity can be traced in literary
and scientific records. The nineteenth century cannot claim to have discovered the
fact, nor can the twentieth century yet claim
to have exhausted the pathology of the
disorder. But it remains true that, for the
ends of administration, the whole history
of the disease before Koch may be blotted out
of our books. Even with the isolation of
the bacillus, the administrative problem was
weighted by a thousand irrelevancies. The
pre-Koch pathology is far from dead. It
still perverts the bedside mind. It is still
repeated in the text-books. It still crowds
the lectures with antiquarian rubbish. It
clouds the mind of the student with useless knowledge. It blocks the way to frank-
ness of outlook and precision of practice.
Curiously, it has faded most rapidly where
the lay mind has had to be convinced. For,
to teach the farmer, or the salesman, or the
butcher, or the dairyman, or the mother of
children, or any of the other innumerable
units that constitute an organised society,
all the delicacies contained in the ancient

theories of a " wasting disease " would have
been a hopeless and futile task. Even the
youngest medical officer of health—fresh,
enthusiastic, full of Virchow and not ignorant
of Darwin—would have been beating his
head against the rocks had he tried to rouse
in the lay mind any interest answering to his
own. Until Koch, the disease was too difficult, too complex, too little understood, to
be taught to any but technically trained
people. But when Koch came, a note of
hope rang round the world. He passed
through the fire of criticism, not scathless,
but carrying with him his cardinal fact—
that where his bacillus was, there also was
tuberculosis. The word tuberculosis passed
from the vagueness of speculative pathology
into the circle of positive science. It was
henceforth to mean something as definite
as gunpowder, or oxygen, or steam. Forthwith, tuberculosis became a doctrine that
the lay mind could grasp. It could be
taught as easily as the multiplication table,
and it could be shown to be as practical.

So far, well. But this alone, though it
excited the hopes of the world and simplified
the duty of the administrator, would not
have secured the growing interest of the
layman. To him a new germ may be an
interesting curiosity ; he will listen to tales

about it ; he will take pride in repeating its
name. But he is nothing if not practical.
If you cannot do him some definite good,
you will tire his interest and you will provoke
him to reaction. Fast on the heels of the
new bacillus came the suggestion that the
disease due to it was no longer hopeless and
incurable. Then the whole world began to
ask for a miracle. It seemed for a time as if
the miracle had happened and the diseased
were to be made whole. The heart sank
when the signs failed. But the miracle had
indeed happened, although the revelation
of it was looked for too soon. Science on the
one hand, and on the other hand Nature, came
once more together, and the open-air treatment became a fact. Meanwhile, science
pushed forward more and more intensively,
until new facts, new methods, new habits of
the organism revealed themselves, and now,
after all, the tuberculin cure of tuberculosis
is no longer a dream of possibilities, but a
definitely established doctrine. The conditions are not so simple as the natural feelings
led us to imagine ; but they are not so complex as to have baffled the patience of research. The day is here when, not as a vague
belief resting on unsolved mysteries, but as a
permissible deduction from ascertained fact,
the forecast of the near future may be—

tuberculosis will be extirpated, or reduced, or, by a simple biological bargain, converted from an enemy to a friend.

So far, again, well. But in the popular mind there was another obstacle. Biology, on the authority of great names, had left us with a crude theory of inheritance. What could it profit that we isolated the bacillus if the personal pedigree were bad ? Did we not hear tales of families swept away, member after member, each when his day came ? Were we not filled with horror at the inherited taint ? Did not the insurance companies, do they not still, base their calculations on the belief that a phthisical inheritance ought to mean a loaded premium ? And in some sense, they are perhaps justified. But the countenance began to lighten and the action to grow athletic when it was, again after long research, made clear that tuberculosis is not inherited—that it is mainly a thing of the environment. It is, in fact, a struggle between two organisms, a lower and a higher. The lower is the invader, the parasite ; but the higher has now in theory become the master. The vague hopes of the earlier days are now planted firmly on a basis of definite inductions. The bacillus can be isolated ; it can be killed ; it can be traced into a thousand by-paths ; it can be stopped at a thousand points of its path from one mouth to another ; it does not pass from generation to generation.

To the administrator, the isolation of the bacillus made the problem simple. To the reformer, the growing belief in the non-inheritance of the disease has offered a new basis of action. The reformer is justified in taking as his objective a possible society of persons immune or immunisable to tuberculosis. The administrator has now to devise the methods of attaining that end.

Ever since Koch's discovery, conviction has been gaining ground that the spread of tuberculosis can be limited by administrative methods. In many parts of Europe and America it has been so limited. There is a good deal of evidence for the proposition that the isolation of phthisical cases has materially reduced the total number of cases. It is true that, for fifty years, the death-rate from phthisis in Britain has fallen year by year until to-day it is only about 50 per cent. of what it was. It has been assumed, without much effort at analysis, that this steady decrease has been the result of improved " general sanitation." Doubtless, general sanitation has contributed much, if under " general sanitation " we include the draining

of soils, the sewering of towns, the improvement in houses, the increase in cleanliness of
habit, and most of all the steady, remorseless,
systematic campaign against infection of
every form. What destroys one infection
destroys another. Incidentally, in our efforts
to limit typhus, typhoid, puerperal fever,
scarlet fever, diphtheria, septicæmia, pyæmia,
and many other infections, we have been
dealing, intimately and in detail, with the
same conditions as the tubercle bacillus
thrives in. In killing typhus and typhoid,
we have, doubtless, without intending it,
killed also tuberculosis, but the tubercle
bacillus is a slowly invading and most persistent parasite. It gets to places that few
other parasites can invade. Everywhere it
finds a nest so easily that it is naturally the
last to be expelled. Precisely because it
kills slowly, it kills most. That is probably
why, when most of the other parasites steadily
fall back before isolation, disinfection, and
protective injections, phthisis needs more
determined and subtle dealing. But, with
every allowance for the insidiousness of this
slow parasite, we are now justified in our
conclusion that by direct attack, as in typhus,
typhoid, scarlet fever, and the others, we shall
be able to reduce the spread of the disease
by securing that the patient shall confine

his infection to himself. To this we are now able to add direct methods of cure. When cure and prevention can, as they ultimately will, work perfectly together, tuberculosis will fall back to the social status of plague and cholera in the western world.

Is tuberculosis of the lungs an infectious disease ? It is. The proofs of its infectivity are overwhelming ; but the methods of its transfer from person to person are infinitely various and difficult to determine. That it is infectious, however, even in the popular sense, is not open to question. The bacillus can be cultivated outside the body ; it can be inoculated into animals, and produces in them the same sequence of signs and symptoms as in human beings. In hundreds of cases, collected by Koch and others, it has been accidentally inoculated into human beings, giving rise to local infection of the glands precisely as in the common untraced infections of glands in children or adults. It has been dried, powdered, and given to guinea-pigs as a dust-inhalation. The result was lung tuberculosis. In 1899, Flügge, by a series of experimental tests, showed " that speaking, coughing, and sneezing produce a thin spray of minute drops which, in the case of tuberculous persons, have been shown

to contain bacilli." Heymann showed that
such drops may be projected to the distance
of a foot and a half from the patient's mouth.
" Out of thirty-five patients experimented
on, fourteen were found to have tubercle-
bacilli - laden drops." Laschtschenko en-
closed a patient in " a glass case for an hour
and a half ; he coughed spontaneously and
also intentionally at intervals, but the amount
of coughing was not extraordinary. In the
glass case were cups containing a weak saline
solution. The contents of these cups were
injected intra-peritoneally (into the abdomen)
into guinea-pigs. Out of nine tests, four gave
positive results. It is thus shown that a
tuberculous patient can spray the surround-
ing area with minute drops containing virulent tubercle bacilli." Flügge showed that
guinea-pigs can be infected by exposing them
to be " coughed at " by tuberculous patients.
All the experiments go to demonstrate that
the moist sputum sprayed from the mouth
of patients in the advanced stages of
the disease are much the most virulently
infectious.

These experimental results are confirmed by
masses of other observations. It matters
nothing whether the material is breathed in
and then swallowed, as Professor St. Clair
Symmers strongly maintains, or inhaled by the

lungs. The practical result is the same. No person capable of estimating the evidence will now withhold assent to the proposition that tuberculosis of the lungs is infectious from person to person. This, on the large scale, is confirmed by the figures so carefully analysed by Dr. Newsholme to exhibit the part that segregation in institutions (workhouses, infirmaries, hospitals, asylums) has played as one of the factors in the decreasing death-rate.

The administrative control of pulmonary phthisis, or tuberculosis of the lungs, is increasing rapidly all over the world. In Scotland, it was provided for, in words, if not by intention, in the Public Health (Scotland) Act, 1897. As that Act contains no definition of infectious disease, the denotation of that term is to be settled by the scientific opinion of the day. What applies to one infection applies to another. By a later Act, certain too stringent clauses of the earlier Act were modified. It can now with truth be said that, without unnecessary hardship to individuals, the full resources of the Public Health Law in Scotland can be brought to bear on every variety of pulmonary tuberculosis. But the administrative value of the statutory provisions was not actively

developed until 1906, when the Local Government Board for Scotland issued a circular on
the administrative control of pulmonary
phthisis. This circular concentrated the mind
of the health authorities on their statutory
obligations, which, hitherto, had been left,
to a great extent, unacknowledged and un-
discharged. Among other things, the Board
recommended that pulmonary tuberculosis
should be added to the list of diseases com-
pulsorily notifiable. There were recommendations, too, on hospitals, on sanatoria,
on disinfection, on dispensaries, and, generally,
on the whole question of pulmonary tuberculosis as affecting the administrative organisations. The response of the localities through
these five years has been extraordinary.

In England, the course of administrative
evolution has been great, but on somewhat
different lines. In 1908, the Local Government
Board of England issued an Order requiring the
notification of all cases of pulmonary tuberculosis that occur in the workhouses, in infirmaries, and among the poor on outdoor relief.
This Order was issued under the same powers
as enable the Local Government Boards of
England, Scotland, and Ireland to deal with
any " epidemic, endemic, or infectious disease,"
including the great international epidemic
diseases—plague, cholera, and yellow fever.

Tuberculosis is to be regarded as an endemic disease. Later, the English Board has issued a second Order requiring notification of pulmonary tuberculosis by all public dispensaries and hospitals in England ; requiring, too, the sanitary authorities to follow up the notifications on certain lines of preventive administration.

Ireland has also taken great strides forward. At the instance of the Irish Local Government Board, an Act was passed enabling the Board to require notification of pulmonary phthisis and to make further provision by hospital and dispensary.

Officially, therefore, the three kingdoms have effectively entered on an administrative campaign against pulmonary tuberculosis. There is, however, nothing to limit administration to tuberculosis of the lungs alone. Every form of tuberculosis will ultimately benefit, and the demand is already heard for more direct dealing with tuberculosis of the bones, of the joints, of the skin ; in a word, " surgical tuberculosis."

The administrative activity shown in Great Britain and Ireland is only part of a world-wide movement. All the nations come together every three years at the International Congress of Tuberculosis, where all the great questions of diagnosis, cure, and adminis-

trative control are discussed and re-discussed.
The policy of the governing bodies, therefore,
cannot any longer be regarded as the hasty
and indiscreet application of abstract ideas
to a practical problem ; it is a well-considered
policy of skilled statesmen, moving slowly
and deliberately in response to ascertained
social demands.

In many localities of Scotland voluntary
notification systems have been tried, and in
some localities they still continue. But experience has shown that voluntary notification is, on the whole, a failure. Now that
the Public Health Act has been adapted to
phthisis, local authorities are much more
ready to add phthisis to the list of the com-
pulsorily notifiable diseases. The following
figures will indicate the rapid rate of progress
now established.

In 1906, not a single health authority of
the whole 313 had adopted compulsory
notification. In 1907, compulsory notification was adopted by 8 health authorities—
4 towns, 4 county districts—representing a
population of 589,698, or 13·2 per cent. of the
population of Scotland. In 1908, the number
of adopting local authorities rose to 10—
5 towns, 5 county districts—representing a
total population of 634,467, or 14·2 per cent.

of the population of Scotland. In 1909, the
number of adopting local authorities rose to
53—30 towns, 23 county districts—representing a total population of 1,150,344, or
26 per cent. of Scotland. In 1910, 82 health
authorities applied the Act—47 towns and
35 county districts—representing a total
population of 2,281,388, or approximately
51 per cent. of the whole population of Scotland. In 1911, up to the end of March, 89
health authorities have applied the Act—
52 towns and 37 county districts—representing a total population of 2,359,154, or
53 per cent. of the whole population of Scotland. The Board's first circular was issued
in 1906. The phenomenal spread of notification has taken place within five years.
In several places the Act has been only tem-
porarily adopted, but it has always been
renewed when the period expired.

These are the facts about notification in
Scotland. In the days before notification
became popular, we heard a great deal about
the probable hardships to individuals, social
ostracism, boycotting, and similar difficulties.
The same has always been said at some stage
about notification of the ordinary infections
Yet no Act works more smoothly than the
Notification Act. Up till now we have
rarely heard of anything but friendly services

to the sick. The stricken people are too eager to find ways of recovering their health to be worried about any sort of social consequences. The experience everywhere is that when treatment, whether much or little, is provided, the claimants never fail to come forward spontaneously. To use words like *ostracise*, *boycotting*, and similar terms of the inexperienced amateur is now a practice long out of date in Scotland. We know better. These are, I am afraid, only the prejudiced phantasies of the unilluminated. They are, however, balanced by the opposite strain of difficulties, namely, the exaggerated fear that the resources of any health authority will be overwhelmed by the claimants for treatment. This, too, is contradicted by experience. As numbers come forward, ways for their reasonable treatment continue to open up. Here a little and there a little, something is being done, and, as time grows older, the administrative pace grows quicker ; for, on the one hand, the public authorities are more and more realising their public duty, and, on the other hand, the private patients are animated more and more by well-founded hopes of recovery. These two tendencies are now in full play, and already, thanks to long and persistent educational efforts, health authorities and patients alike are swept forward by a social momentum that nothing will arrest or divert.

Hitherto men have rested the significance of the notification of phthisis on the fact that it is an infectious disease. This is important, but it does not explain the real significance of notification. This significance lies rather in the fact that, when a disease is once notified, the patients must be dealt with, not in the mass, but as individual cases. In the days when we knew only of the existence of masses of disease—crowds of cases of typhus, of typhoid, of smallpox, of scarlet fever—naturally preventive measures took the form of improving the general environment, the drains, the water-supply, the sites of houses, and the like. But as soon as individual cases came to be notified, each case had to be dealt with on its own special merits, isolated, and treated according to its needs. That is what notification has done for the infectious diseases. That is what it is now doing for phthisis. We are long past the stage when we stop at general improvement of the environment. We are now well into the stage when we must deal with the individual case and his individual environment That is why notification is important. It enables the health authority to bring the full

force of an improved environment to bear
on the specific needs of the individual patient.

What has somewhat amazed, if not amused,
me in this whole movement is the curious
paradox that, in all other infectious diseases,
such as typhoid, scarlet fever, etc., it is con-
sidered right and necessary for the Health
Authority to deal with the individual patient ;
but, in pulmonary phthisis, many maintain
that we should leave the individual patient
alone, and deal only with the environment.
The death-rate, it is alleged, is going down
" of itself." Improve housing, improve food,
improve the environment generally, but leave
the private patient to the private doctor.
Apparently some men are more or less
satisfied with the way the death-rate is going
down. I am not. It is going down, but not
fast enough.

And it is not going down of its own accord,
or from any mysterious influence of the
Time Spirit. It is going down because we are
putting it down. It has been going down
ever since the serious work of sanitation in
Scotland began, say, seventy years ago. It
continues to go down because the medical
men are getting to understand phthisis
better, because they are diagnosing it earlier,
because they are helping forward the im-

provement of the surroundings, because they are letting fresh air into the houses, because they are reducing the consumption of alcohol, because they are beginning to understand dietetics better. It is going down, too, because the Medical Officers of Health are, day in, day out, pushing forward the operation of every variety of health machinery,—the cleansing of houses, the disinfection of houses and persons and clothing, the steadily increasing isolation of as many varieties of acute infection as are likely to benefit by that measure, and, in a word, every proceeding that places the individual patient in a better environment, permanent or temporary,—so increasing the personal resistance and reducing the complications of the acute infections.

It is going down, too, because the Sanitary Inspectors and Borough Engineers maintain a ruthless attack on damp houses, defective drains, defective ventilation, dirty rooms, dirty people, dirty clothing, over-crowding,—so reducing on every hand the chances of contracting any infection, tuberculosis among the rest.

It is going down, too, because the Inspectors of Poor and the Parish Councils are steadily strengthening their grip of this primary cause of pauperism.

But the pace of the down-going of the death-

rate is still very slow.   So long as we can say
that in Scotland alone nearly six thousand
people die every year of phthisis, this one
form of tuberculosis, the pressure of administrative measures should never slack.   And, so
long as I have an administrative breath to
draw, it never shall slack.   The belief that the
death-rate is going down of itself and rapidly
enough, looks like the special pleading of the
interested or the fatuity of the fatalist.   The
belief is an erroneous belief.

Before I end this chapter, I cannot resist
the temptation to make a remark on certain
" red herrings " that are persistently drawn
across the administrative scent.   I call them
" red herrings " somewhat disrespectfully,
because I have repeatedly found that they
are offered, not as a reason for doing something positive on the special line suggested,
but to prevent any one from doing anything
positive on any line whatever.

For instance, it is said, phthisis is a Housing question.   Undoubtedly it is a Housing
question.   So is typhoid fever.   But the
quickest way to get at the house is to deal
with the patient in the house.   That is what
our Housing Acts, and our Public Health
Acts, and, above all, our Town Planning
Acts are there for.   For my part, I should

like to see every health authority in Britain
rise to the great height of the opportunities
it now has to make every house, every hamlet,
every village, every small town, every great
town, serve to the full the ends of business,
health, and beauty. But the direct attack
on phthisis will still have to go on. For
phthisis is much more than a Housing question.
It is an Infantile question. To meet that, we
have our Notification of Births Act and the
Children Act. These contain immense powers,
and all the powers are powers of dealing with
the individual. The crop of health visitors,
voluntary and official, is the answer to the
children question. It is also a School Child
question. The answer to that is the system
of medical inspection, now happily established over the length and breadth of the
kingdom. If it should finally appear that the
great period of personal infection is, as von
Behring maintains, the period of infancy,
the shortest way to bring assistance to mother
and child is to deal individually with both.
If it should be established, as is probable,
that practically every child is, in one degree
or another, at some time or another, infected
with tuberculosis, and if it be true that a
limited dose acts in some measure as an
immunising agency, it is all the more impera-
tive that we should deal with the individual

child and his personal environment, and so, by clearing away all sources of major infection, keep down the dose to the relatively harmless minimum. Phthisis is also a Food question. The answer to that is our elaborate Food Acts, our power of dealing with meat and milk. If milk is the chief factor of infection, the shortest way to the guilty dairy is to start from the infected child. All our dairy regulations and milk acts have arisen out of the clinical physician's demand for an explanation of this or that infectious disease. But phthisis is also a Factory question. The answer to that is the unremitting enforcement of the Factory and Workshop Acts. And so, through every other one of the many relations of administrative control, we must work the administrative machinery we have or devise machinery more suitable. The whole campaign must go forward at once. For all these special questions are strung on a single thread —the thread of the individual life. We have talked long enough about the big things. We are now in the full tide of the little duties that make the big things possible. In Scotland we need no more legislation for the moment. We need first to work for all it is worth the legislation we have. In Scotland we have taken our own line, and we intend to keep it. We have shown that the powers of our statutes are simple and effective. All we require is the wish and the will to work them. The facts I have given are proof that neither the wish nor the will is wanting. To every man that wants to live, we would offer the chance to live

CHAPTER X

THE INTERNATIONAL INFECTIONS—PLAGUE, CHOLERA, AND YELLOW FEVER

WHEN plague came to Glasgow eleven years ago, there were sceptics to question the identity of the disease. True, the first cases emerged under a curious guise. A child and its grandmother, living in the same house, had sickened suddenly. Four days later the child died of " zymotic enteritis " (a form of diarrhœa). Two days later the grandmother died of " acute gastro-enteritis." In both cases a " wake " was held. The grandmother was buried on the third day after death. Her husband sickened the day after the burial ; but it was not until fifteen days later that he was admitted to hospital as "enteric fever." Other sicknesses, not at first known to be related to the same focus, rapidly appeared. Three cases were provisionally diagnosed as "enteric fever." The medical attendants, however, were not satisfied; but they knew the cases were infectious and wished to bring them to the knowledge of the health authority. On admission to the hospital, these cases were carefully examined. The physician concluded that "the patients were suffering from Bubonic Plague, although they were inhabitants of Glasgow and there was no known case of Bubonic Plague in Britain."

So the long record of two centuries and a half was broken. The identity of the ancient plague of London and the modern plague in Glasgow was proved. And the proof came of the insight of a skilled physician, who, though he had never seen plague, kept an "open sense." His first conjecture was confirmed within a few minutes. Within a few days, it was absolutely established by an independent expert. The instantaneous conjecture was thus verified; but it was the interest of a million people to discredit it. To those familiar with the hundreds of thousands, even the millions of deaths, that every year take place in India, such an attitude must seem curious. But I remember as if it were yesterday how the excitement of the event spread everywhere and evoked everywhere the same comments. The diagnosis was a triumph of medicine and bacteriology. The physician quite understood that on the view he took of this microscopic germ would depend the closing of the port, the interruption of the shipping, the establishing of the strictest scrutiny at every continental port, the institution of a laborious survey of the infected area of the city, the searching out of contacts, the cleansing of houses and stores, the hunting of rats, and a thousand other administrative activities in Glasgow and the other cities of Britain. Yet the diagnosis was made and announced. It stood the test. And every fresh case confirmed it. Experts from East and West confirmed it. The subsequent history of Glasgow itself confirmed it, for plague appeared again a year or two later in rats and in men.

The discovery of an identity in circumstances so different as those of London in 1665 and those of Glasgow in 1899 has an intellectual interest all its own. But to Glasgow, directly and indirectly, the discovery meant the loss of thousands upon thousands of pounds. Plague was still a terror, though it was a terror under control. But the attitude of the official organisation towards it was the attitude of

a master.   The city, by the persistent application of her vast resources and her elaborate
sanitary police, did, with the general mind
all alert and open, succeed in keeping the
treacherous disease within narrow limits.   By
good fortune wakes were not obsolete ; therefore the quick succession of cases revealed
the seriousness of the situation.   But for
this fortunate bad social habit, the city might
have had to reckon its cases, not by groups
of one and two, but by groups of tens and
hundreds.   The original case was never, I
believe, discovered.   This is not strange to
those that know how casual life is among the
people affected.   Care sits lightly on them
when they are sober, and when they are
drunk memory is the memory of dreams, and
experiences vanish like morning gossamer on
the hillsides.

This and other outbreaks in Europe led
to the revision of the Venice Convention,
which then regulated the international health
relations of nearly all the European states.
The part that rats played in the spread of
plague had been made familiar by the Report
of the Royal Commission on Indian Plague.
In the Agreement of Paris, 1903, the modern
knowledge of plague was incorporated.   By
this agreement plague, cholera, and yellow

fever are to-day regulated all over the world.

Of these three not one is endemic in Britain. They normally enter this country by a large seaport. As all the leading seaports are customs ports, the customs officers form the first line of defence. Any vessel from any foreign port that is infected with plague, cholera, or yellow fever, is challenged by the boarding officer, who asks certain definite questions from the master, who, in turn, must, under heavy penalties, answer correctly. If any case of plague, or suspected plague, or any case of illness exists on board, the customs officer stops the vessel. He reports the facts to the Medical Officer of Health for the port. He, in turn, must visit and examine within twelve hours. From the time he boards the vessel until he completes his examination, he has full control of the ship and every person on it. If he finds a case of plague on board, he has full powers to order the ship to anchor in the place provided, to remove the case to hospital, to remove suspected cases, to disinfect, to retain suspected cases until the nature of the disease is ascertained. He also takes the name, address, and destination of every person that wishes to leave the ship, forwards the information to the officials at the destination named, and thus secures that all along the course a certain amount of supervision is exercised.   Sailors, as a rule, are ready enough to go to hospital rather than leave the port ; but the freedom of movement now accorded to passengers and crews has been evolved out of a long experience of the tendency to concealment and evasion.   Concealment and evasion, however, are much commoner among passengers than among crews.   In six years of pretty active port life, I never found a master or officer that was not quite ready to reveal every important fact of the voyage. The shipping companies are only too anxious to keep themselves right with the law.   If, however, an infected ship enters harbour without suspicion, the Medical Officer of Health still has a reserve power.   If he suspects that the ship is infected, or comes from an infected port, he may examine the vessel and take all measures necessary to make it safe.   The number of ships, however, that escape the lynx eyes of the customs officers is small.

In British ports, quarantine, as formerly understood, is not legally required and is not practised.   Every object of quarantine is obtained by the method I have sketched. Such quarantine as is practised at all, is carried out on shore ; the ship is set free at the earliest possible moment, and thus the interests of the commercial community are little injured. For the carrying out of the Agreement of Paris, each country has its own special regulations ; but these, in nearly all the signatory countries, are now much the same as in Britain. Everywhere, provision is now made for dealing with rats. These are a greater danger than human beings. How great the danger is the appearance of plague among rats in the east of England last year has made manifest. It is known that in India rat plague precedes human plague. As rat plague now exists in Britain, the precautions against human plague, no less than against rat plague, have to be all the more stringent.

The Agreement of Paris, based as it is on actual experience of plague in the West, is more adaptable to western conditions than any previous agreement. Five days after the death or isolation of the last known case of plague, a commercial port may once more be declared free. Usually, cases are under isolation as suspects for some days before plague can be demonstrated. The result is that commerce is not now liable to be seriously interrupted. How much this means to the comity of nations only those can understand that have had to stop, even for an hour, one small tributary of the great stream of international commerce.

Plague, in spite of every precaution, scientific and administrative, continues to kill its millions in India, to spread steadily over East and West, and to-day it leaves no continent unaffected. It is in the strictest sense an international epidemic. Any hour may bring fresh cases to our shores, but the probability of a widespread epidemic in Britain is not great ; the scouting is too alert, the administrative machinery too mobile, the general interest too informed, the general fear too intense. Imported cases, outbreaks, little epidemics there may be, but an epidemic on the scale of the great plague of London is not likely to occur in any of the western or northern countries of Europe.

In the last fifteen years plague has been well " worked over " scientifically. Preventive serums and vaccines have been devised. Their success more than justifies their use ; but the problem of prevention in Eastern countries needs more than curative serums. The sanitary conditions of the hot countries present difficulties unknown to the West. The rat population of Calcutta is said to be greater than the very great human population.

The rat is among the most prolific of the rodents. He goes everywhere and lives. Up till now, he has defied every civilisation. He is the menace of empires. Malaria, it is suggested, came from Egypt to Greece with the slaves. Plague goes all over the world with the rat. He has his defenders, who count him a good scavenger. He has his detractors, who count him an expensive luxury. Perhaps he has a beneficent place in nature ; but, for the moment, he is an enemy of mankind.

Plague is spread by the rat. Cholera is spread by water.

Briefly, cholera is a form of diarrhœa— violent, contagious, and rapidly fatal ; attended with agonising pains in the digestive organs, cramps all over the body, and great depression. The disease lies dormant for about two days after it is first caught ; it then strikes suddenly, and often in the night, and then, within a limited number of hours, it runs towards death or recovery. Cholera, thus marked in its main features, is due to a specific poison. Koch maintained that the poison is from a specific microbe, viz., the Comma Bacillus. This he discovered in several places, viz., in the discharges of cholera patients, in the bowels after death, and in cisterns of drinking-water that he knew to be infected. He isolated the bacillus and cultivated it. The bacillus is an unquestionable fact ; it may be seen in any pathologist's laboratory. But Koch cannot be held to have demonstrated its causative action in cholera, though recent research tends to confirm his view. But, whatever the germ be, the poison is a specific poison ; it produces a distinct and invariable train of symptoms ; it is carried by water, by clothing, by food, by every variety of human intercourse. It had its original home probably in India. It became fully recognised at the beginning of last century ; time and again it has spread westward, and towards the end of the nineteenth century it was once more in force within two or three days' journey of our shores. Occasional cases have come across the Continent since 1892 ; but there has been no serious outbreak in Great Britain.

" In the nineteenth - century annals of pestilence," writes Hirsch, " the year 1817 stands as one charged with fatality to the human race. It was in that year there began the epidemic extension over India of a disease which had previously been known only as an endemic in a few districts of the country ; in that and the following year it overran

the whole peninsula ; in a short time it
crossed the borders of its native territory
in all directions, penetrated in its farther
progress to almost every part of the habitable
globe, and thus acquired the character of a
world-wide pestilence, which has repeatedly
since then entered on its devastating cam-
paigns, and has claimed its many millions of
victims." Cholera, thus breaking its primitive bounds, has come westward and spread
over the world four times during the nineteenth century. The first time was from
1817 to 1823, when it all but crossed the
frontiers of the European Continent. The
second time was in 1826. In this year it
broke out in India ; before the end of 1830
" the pestilence had obtained an extensive
footing on Russian soil " ; from Russia it
came to Germany, and from Germany in
1831 it came to Great Britain. The places
first affected were Sunderland, Newcastle,
Gateshead, Haddington (1832), Musselburgh,
Edinburgh, Glasgow, Belfast, Cork. " Thus
in the course of the year it spread over a great
part of Britain, following the commercial
highways chiefly, and the coast routes and
rivers ; while the mountainous parts of
the country were little visited by it, and the
Scottish Highlands not at all."—(Hirsch.)
This great epidemic ended in 1838, and for

ten years Europe was free from cholera. The third great epidemic began in 1846. In 1847 it was in Russia, Astrakhan, along the Volga, and round the shores of the Sea of Azov. In 1848, it appeared in England and Scotland. Among the Scotch towns visited were Edinburgh, Glasgow, and Dumfries. The fourth great epidemic began in 1863. As in the other epidemics, the European countries were nearly all visited. In Scotland, during 1865, there were 1170 cholera deaths. In 1873, cholera was still common in many parts of the Continent, and at many seaports in Britain cases were landed ; but in Britain itself the disease did not spread inland.

All through the history of these epidemics one tracks the disease to the great seaports everywhere. These are the natural landing-places of such an enemy.

The last epidemic of cholera in Scotland undoubtedly hastened the passing of the Public Health Act of 1867,—an Act full of sagacious and advanced provisions. The scare resulted in a small crop of separate cholera hospitals, which have almost entirely stood empty ever since they were built. But the impulse so generated has been beneficial in every direction. It taught the people the need of pure water. It prepared the way for the great reform of 1889, when public health was transferred bodily from the rural Poor Law Authorities to a special Health Authority with a larger area. The continued menace of cholera, assisted by outbreaks of typhoid fever, has worked a marvellous reform in water supplies all over Britain. The preventive health service has been going on for these twenty years un-relentingly. It has been steadily removing from every corner of the country the condi-tions that would favour a widespread out-break of cholera. The danger of such an outbreak, though less to-day than even twenty years ago, is far from small. It can be met only by active administration.

Of the three international epidemic diseases, yellow fever remains. But in the colder climates yellow fever is not a danger. It may be imported, but it cannot live ; for the mosquito that spreads it is not a native of the cold climates. But the disease is still a great danger to many countries of the world. As the problems of malaria centre round one mosquito, the problems of yellow fever centre round another. Either this mosquito must be destroyed, or a remedy found to make its specific injection harmless. Of this there seems to be no doubt. Experiments such as this have been carried out :—Mos-

quitoes were "fed on the blood of yellow
fever patients not less than twelve days
previously." They were then permitted to
bite ten persons that had never had the
disease and were in no way protected against
it.   Of the ten bitten, eight developed the
disease.   Apparently the mosquito needs some
twelve days to become infectious.   If he bites
to-day, taking with him the germ from the
blood of the patient, he is harmless until the
germ develops within him.   This takes twelve
days.   If he then bites a healthy person, he
conveys the disease.

Here once more we are on the borderland
of biology.   The plague germ has the rat
and the rat flea ;   the cholera germ has the
water ;   the yellow fever germ has its own
mosquito.   To save the afflicted peoples preventive medicine must upset those " balances
of nature."   Man must fit his environment
to himself.   It is curious that, when those
great diseases are in question, nothing is heard
about heredity, or the danger of preserving
the unfit, or the sacrilege of not permitting
the socially rejected to work out their own
salvation by natural selection.   Why do we
hear so little in this strain ?   Because plague,
cholera, yellow fever, malaria, are none of
them respecters of persons.   They attack the
strong and robust as readily as they attack

the feeble. They kill without discrimination. If they were left to roam the world unrestricted, the remnants that would survive would be, indeed, more " fit " to continue in a world flooded with those four diseases, but they would not thereby be the " fittest " for the work of great civilisations. When strong men have to fight against foreign enemies like these, they have no time to concern themselves with fears about heredity. It is only when faced with familiar destroyers like tuberculosis, or measles, or poisonous trades, that they lend an easy ear to proposals for letting the " unfit " die. They yield less to logic, perhaps, than to psychology. It is this that makes the health service scrutinise with the most active scepticism everything that touches the theory of heredity, when that theory is used to foster an attitude of impotence in the face of preventable disease. And this attitude, I regret to think, seems to attract only too readily the non-administrative speculators in heredity.

CHAPTER XI

OTHER PREVENTABLE DISEASES

THE infections, though not all equally preventable, are pre-eminently preventable diseases. But there are others. How great the mass of them is could be learned only from a careful scrutiny of the whole list of diseases. Here I offer only a few gross indications.

Long ago, in his book on *The Hygiene, Diseases, and Mortality of Occupations*, Dr. J T. Arlidge gave a carefully elaborated analysis of the occupational diseases. He first classified occupations, following the lead of Dr. Ogle and Dr. Farr. He then set himself to a systematic study of the correlative diseases. Not an important trade escaped his observation. But he laid special stress on the dust diseases,—the diseases arising out of the dusty occupations. Many manufactures generate dust. There are mineral dusts,—metallic, as in file-making, or razor-grinding ; non-metallic, as in coal-mining, tin-mining, flint-working, slate-quarrying, china-painting, and a number of others. Then there are dusts of organic origin,—some of them vegetable, such as the dust of cotton-manufacturing, cotton-cloth sizing, flax-work, linen-manufacturing, seed-crushing, tobacco-manufacturing. And there are organic dusts of animal origin, as in cloth and shoddy manufacture, hosiery manufacture, wool-sorting. Then there is the large range of occupations where poisonous materials are dealt with. There are others where noxious vapours are constantly encountered. There are others where the temperature is excessive ; others where the strain, pressure, and friction are too prolonged. In a book of nearly six hundred large crowded pages, Dr. Arlidge professed to give only a condensed sketch of the occupational diseases.

This volume had much to do with improvements both in legislation and in adminis-tration. Commissions on the dangerous trades have gone into great detail in examining the precise processes of manufacture, the prob-able and actual effects on health, and the amount of illness due to the particular trades. On the basis of such inquiries, the Home Office, which is the central authority for the administration of the Factory Acts, has for years set itself systematically to reduce the occupational diseases. Not a month passes but some fresh or revised regulation is issued to meet some hitherto unregulated cause of disease or death. The mass of these regula-tions is very great ; but not one is enacted

without an elaborate inquiry into the whole
conditions of the given trade and the given
process. If one would know the vast area
covered by the Medical Department of the
Home Office, he has only to glance at the
yearly and occasional reports of the Chief
Factory Inspector, Dr. Arthur Whitelegge,
C.B. There is not a dangerous or unwhole-
some trade that he and his Department do
not know. There is no department of central
administration more vitally in touch with
the environment of labour.

The rapid expansion of industry, the continued improvement in methods, the increased
demand for more healthy conditions, all
combine to make the occupational diseases
more and more a subject for special study.
In a book on *Dangerous Trades*, edited by
Professor Thomas Oliver, will be found nearly
a thousand pages of standard information in
sixty chapters, not only on the hygiene of
the special trades, but on the special diseases
and general questions arising out of them.
The work includes among its experts, factory
inspectors, medical officers of health, statisticians, and others familiar with special
processes or diseases.

To take but one or two illustrations. Of
all the poisonous metals, lead, because it is
so widely used, is probably the most destruc-

tive. Lead-mining, lead-smelting, the manufacture of red-lead, of white-lead, and
manufactures where these substances
are used, may all lead to lead-poison-
ing. " Lead is a subtle poison," writes
Professor Oliver. " Most of its salts have in
small doses no unpleasant taste or odour,
they are very soluble, and they produce their
baneful effects sometimes in such an insidious
manner that the health of the operative
becomes so gradually undermined that he is
often precipitated into a serious illness without
any warning. In most instances, however,
there are prodromata (preliminary symptoms),
for lead causes colic or severe pain in the
abdomen." The effect of lead on women is in
the highest degree evil. It seriously interferes with the maternal powers. " Children
of female lead-workers almost invariably die
of convulsions shortly after birth or during the
first twelve months. If a child is the offspring of parents both of whom are lead-
workers, it is puny and ill-nourished, and is
either born dead, or dies a few hours after
birth." Lead is even more dangerous. It
not only kills the offspring ; it destroys " for
the time being the child-bearing powers of
women." But why continue ? To describe
fully the effects of lead alone would take much
more than the present volume. Let one

further quotation be enough. " It is upon pregnant women that the metal exercises its worst effects. . . . When a white-lead worker becomes pregnant it is almost impossible for her to go to the end of term if she continues to follow her employment. . . . In the liver and kidneys of still-born children of female lead-workers . . . there were found minute quantities of lead. . . . Mrs. H., age thirty-five, worked in a white-lead factory for six years, before which she had four children born at full time. Since going to the lead-works she has had nine miscarriages in succession and no living child." These facts can be added to indefinitely. If, as some social critics assert, the effect of preventive medicine is to preserve the unfit, here is a fair case for testing the view. But if the high infant mortality in certain industries is to be a test of the unfitness, let the infants at least start fair. Let them come into the world at the instance of healthy nature, not under the expulsive power of lead.

But though lead-working is the most strik-ing, it is not the only poisonous industry. The manufacture of arsenic contributes its share to the disabled. So does the manufacture of rubber. " Girls have told me that on leaving the factory at night they have simply staggered home. . . . Prolonged exposure to the vapour of bisulphide induces an enfeeblement of the intelligence that recalls the mental weakness of chronic alcoholic inebriety."

Or take this of mercurial poisoning: " The worker becomes pale and loses his appetite. He frequently has headache, giddiness, and transitory pains in the limbs. The muscles of the face twitch, the fingers tremble when spread out, and the tongue is also tremulous when protruded. The mental condition undergoes change. Workers assured of their skill become shy and nervous, especially when watched." The teeth are affected. " Chronic mercurial poisoning does not frequently lead directly to death. It appears to lower the vitality of the tissues markedly, and Kussmaul calls attention to the frequency with which mercurial workers die of phthisis."

Of dust as a cause of occupation disease, Professor Oliver says: " Were it not for dust, fume, or gas, there would be little or no disease of occupation except such as might be caused by infection, the breathing of air poisoned by the emanations of fellow-workmen, and exposure to cold after working in over-heated rooms." He considers that dust plays such a prominent part in the causation of disease that it needs a discussion by itself. The coal miner's lung is familiar at an early stage to every medical student. The steel grinder's lung is common knowledge. But there are also skin diseases arising from certain kinds of dust. These may vary from simple irritation to inflammation, pustules, and ulcers. In some dust trades, the nails suffer. In others, the irritating dust affects the bowel.

These illustrations are enough to point the lesson. The prevention of all these diseases is not only theoretically possible ; it is entirely practicable. Partly, it may be secured by improving the conditions of the manufactures, and this is the object of the stringent regulations everywhere obtaining. Partly, it must assume the co-operation of the worker, and for this also the regulations provide. But familiarity breeds indifference. The result is that, in spite of every precaution and enforcement, the occupational diseases of the dangerous trades will for years to come constitute an appreciable item in the disease roll.

Let us leave this and look to another set of facts. If the diseases named in an earlier chapter are carefully followed out into their individual conditions, many of them will be found entirely preventable. In a volume on the *Prevention of Disease*, translated from the German some years ago, and containing a pointed introduction by Dr. Timbrell Bulstrode, the whole field of medical and surgical diseases has been carefully studied specifically from the standpoint of prevention. " With the rapid growth and diffusion of knowledge as to the prevention of disease," writes Dr. Bulstrode, " the physician will be asked in an ever-increasing degree how the onset of certain pathological conditions may be prevented ; and although he may not, at present, always be in a position to indicate the lines which may be followed, there may, I think, be little doubt that the subject of individual prophylaxis (protective prevention) will occupy an important place in medicine in the near future." With this opinion every member of the preventive medical service will agree. Not until one works carefully through the groups of diseases here studied can he even partially realise how much of current disease can either by early direction or by early treatment be either postponed or prevented. And we do not refer to prevention of the infectious diseases, but to the prevention of heart disease, by judicious nurture in youth and moderate living as life advances ; prevention of digestive diseases, by the careful study of foods and moderation in their use ; prevention of children's diseases, by careful nurture in infancy, systematic inspection and supervision in childhood, attention to teeth, food, and sleep ; prevention of nervous and mental diseases, by the regulation of life and the avoidance of excesses.

Of the special senses there needs only a word—the eye, the ear, the throat, the nose, the teeth, the skin, have all been so fully studied, they are all so important economically, that the great majority of our population realise the need for care in the prevention of their diseases and for immediate cure if disease supervenes. The Medical Inspection of School Children secures the necessary administrative acceleration.

It is, therefore, fully established that out of the many classes of disease many are preventable, partly by improving the general conditions of life, partly by bringing to bear on the individual case the resources of knowledge. The mass of preventable disease is so great that it more than justifies the preventive service evoked by its existence. It does more. It justifies in every person the mental attitude that, in any individual case of sickness or disablement, leads the observer always to ask first—is it preventable ?

There is, of course, the necessary residuum

that no knowledge has yet enabled us to prevent. These are problems of the future. But, meanwhile, every medical service, official and voluntary, is grossly overloaded in the effort to provide even for the coarser diseases that spring from the evil environments of industry. Of the efforts to prevent fatigue and to develop personal resources by an adapted personal hygiene, I say nothing ; they are swamped, except among the leisured. If you would judge how the " pressure of life " tells in the heavier trades, procure and study Dr. Arthur Newsholme's recent report on Infant and Child Mortality. It is said by one writer that " the consequences of that pressure are prevented from producing effects that are of selection value." Dr. Newsholme shows that the " selection value " in the indiscriminate death-dealing of the heavy industries is mostly, if not entirely, mythical. In the counties where the deaths of infants under one year are greatest, there also the deaths of children from one to five and five to ten years are greatest. Any " selection value " that the correlation method reveals is practically nothing, except, doubtfully, for children of the second year. The facts about lead are eloquent of the reason why. Surely it is our first duty to provide an environment that is not certain to kill. We can then take up at leisure those interesting speculations on " selection value." The number of men, women and children incidentally saved for a few years more from death or disablement will not, even if labelled " unfit," seriously affect our social resources.

CHAPTER XII

THE HYGIENICS OF A STAPLE FOOD—MILK

SHALL I, with Mr. Upton Sinclair, fast for ten days and recover on milk and oranges ? Shall I, with Professor Chittenden of Yale, keep my nutrition down to the limits of physiological economy ? Or shall I, with Sir James Crichton-Browne, keep a big excess-margin for contingencies ? Shall I, with Mr. Bernard Shaw, cease eating my fellow-creatures ? Shall I, with Dr. Haig, displace the meat and tea poisons by milk and cheese ? Shall I, with Sydney Smith and his Edinburgh Reviewers, cultivate learning on a little oatmeal ? Or, not to omit a great name from the ever-lengthening chain of dietetic specialists, shall I, under Metchnikoff, the director of the New Hygiene, stop the disease of old age by a diet of soured milk ?

These are questions the modern man puts to himself. Whomsoever he selects from the multitude of skilled counsellors, he will not find one that forbids him milk or the products of milk. Milk, too, is the staple food of infants. Whatever happens to meat, milk will maintain its place ; for the children must be fed. For adults, too, it is practically as indispensable and, as time proceeds, will become increasingly a necessity. In every country in the world, milk has risen in dietetic importance. This is why I select it as a type of the food environment.

The problem of the milk-supply is : To bring to the consumer clean, harmless, palatable cow's milk. By clean, I mean free from adventitious impurities, such as sand, dust, cobwebs, cow-dung, hairs, epithelial scales, and the like. By harmless, I mean not capable of producing any disease, infectious or other. By palatable, I mean not so altered from the natural flavour of wholesome milk as to disgust. Other qualities of milk are equally important, from other points of view. For example, the percentage of butter-fat may be more important than the absolute freedom from dirt ; or, again, fat may be of less importance

than the readiness to decompose. But those
qualities are only indirectly, not directly,
questions for hygienics ; because hygienics,
which here practically means the scientific
care of the human environment, concerns
itself with the reduction in number of abnormal factors. Dirt, disease, and the conse-
quent decompositions of milk may destroy
it as a possible human food, so throwing it out
of relation to the physiological needs. These
three, therefore, it is the first duty of hygienics
to eliminate. Practically, therefore, the problem is how to eliminate dirt and disease, how
to prevent unintended decompositions, and
how, thus, to preserve in its full physiological
relations, a food of immense value. I assume
that milk is a highly important factor in the
food environment of our present highly
complicated society ; that our present methods
of providing the consumer with milk are full
of defects ; that the rectification of these
defects is an entirely practical enterprise.

Under dirt, I include all the non-pathogenic
germs ; for these, though they do indirectly
encourage specific diseases, are not individually associated with any particular disease.
They affect seriously the " keeping " qualities
of milk. They have, therefore, pre-eminently
a bearing on commercial, and, by consequence,

on practical management. They are the pest of the small or the town dairy and the minor shopkeeper. They are the quint-essence of uncleanness. They are, however, in part useful in the production of milk pro-ducts; but in " market " milk, as it goes forth for consumption *as* milk, they are nothing less than destructive ferments. The germs, or micro-organisms, I mean, are mainly these : the lactic ferments (including special bacilli, micrococci, and streptococci, in many varieties), *bacillus coli communis* (in some of its " races "), the casein ferments, the blue milk bacilli, the red milk bacilli, yellow milk bacilli, bitter milk bacilli, the organisms that produce slimy milk, or stringy, or soapy milk. Besides these, there are the yeasts and other moulds.

To protect milk from most of these is not very difficult ; but the care necessary is more than will ever be systematically taken by any but the most scrupulous dairyman. In the cleanest cowsheds I have ever seen, where, too, the cows were well-groomed and looked it, the chances of germ pollution were more than could be readily calculated. There are always at least the following germ-yielding conditions : Dry hay or other fodder, dust from roofs, dust from floors, moulds, dried excreta, decomposing urine, the micro-organisms of the cow's hide, the innumerable germs of ordinary water, the repeated contacts with human hands and clothing. The cows lie down clean ; they rise up dirty.

To watch the milking of cows is to watch a process of unscientific inoculation of a pure (or almost pure) medium with unknown quantities of unspecified germs. Perhaps feeding is just over, or the cows are in fresh from the field ; or, as in town cowsheds, they were in some fields six months ago, and have never seen clear skylight again. In comes the milker, man or woman, slaps the cow's buttock to make her rise. The milkstool is placed, taken from some dirty corner of the cowshed. A few squirts of the teat, or of two teats, are given as a preliminary encouragement to the cow and a convenient lubrication for the fingers. Incidentally, the first squirts may help to clear out any micro-organisms that lodge in the ducts. The hands may be clean—or not. The clothes may be newly washed—or not. The nose, the mouth, the eyes, the ears, the face generally, the hair, may all have been specially cleaned just before—or not. Whoever knows the meaning of aseptic surgery must feel his blood run cold when he watches, even in imagination, the thousand chances of germ inoculation. From cow to cow the milker goes, taking with

her (or him) the stale epithelium of the last
cow, the particles of dirt caught from the
floor, the hairs, the dust, and the germs that
adhere to them. Meanwhile, what with
switching of cows' tails, what with stamping
of feet, the cowshed is in a state of persistent
agitation. The cows are feeding. The im-
prisoned dust of the dry fodder is scattered
to the air currents. Meanwhile, too, the
other milkers are collecting the milk. They
perspire. They transfer the milk from pail
to can. They leave the total to gather more
germs and dust. Perhaps, the moderately
careful dairyman sieves the milk roughly
from the pail ; but the sieve is not such as to
enmesh any but the major particles. Everywhere, throughout the whole process of milking, the perishable, superbly nutrient liquid
receives its repeated sowings of germinal and
non-germinal dirt. In an hour or two, its
population of triumphant lives is a thing
imagination boggles at.

And this in good dairies. What must it be
where the cows are never groomed, where
udders are never washed, where teats are never
rubbed, where the cowsheds are never even
approximately cleaned, where ventilators are
never open, where the dung is a stale heap at
the cowshed door, where the pigs are a few
feet away, where cobwebs are ancient and

heavy, where the ammoniacal emanations of decomposing urine nip the eyes, where hands are only by accident all washed, where heads are only occasionally cleaned, where spittings (tobacco or other) are not infrequent, where the milker may be a chance-comer from some filthy slum,—where, in a word, the various dirts of the civilised human are, at every hand, reinforced by the inevitable dirts of the domesticated cow ?

Are these exaggerations ? They are not. I could name, for town and county, many admirable cowsheds where these conditions are, in greater or less degree, normal. But a general statement of germ-yielding conditions were incomplete without some quantitative confirmation. Here are a few figures from reliable sources :—

Dr. Edward von Freudenreich says : " In Berne I have found on an average 160,000 to 320,000 bacteria per cubic inch in fresh milk ; while Cnopf in Munich estimates the number at 960,000 to 1,600,000 per cubic inch, *i.e.* thirty-three to fifty-six millions per pint." Again, he found that a " sample of milk containing 153,000 bacteria per cubic inch," on being kept at a temperature of 59° F., had, after an hour, 539,750 per cubic inch ; after four hours, 680,000 ; after nine hours, 2,040,000 ; after twenty-five hours, 85,000,000.

In other instances, the increase was even more striking, the temperature being higher. By the time milk usually reaches the consumer in this country, it is certain to contain some millions of germs in each cubic centimetre. Mr. H. L. Russell, of the University of Wisconsin Agricultural Experiment Station, found that " a gelatine plate exposure made in the stalls during the feeding showed that over 160,000 organisms were deposited in a minute on an area covered by an ordinary milk pail."

So much for germinal dirt. Non-germinal dirt has less significance in itself; for its principal effects are essentially those of the adhering germs, and these effects have already been generally indicated. Yet the dirt, apart from the germs, is not unimportant either in amount or in kind. The consumer wishes to consume milk approximately as it comes from the cow. What I have already stated demonstrates how difficult it is, by current methods, to obtain such milk; but to realise how much the dirt, germinal and non-germinal, amounts to, one must examine actual specimens.

Let one spend half a day or so at a creamery where, say, 6000 to 10,000 gallons of milk are dealt with between 7 a.m. and 4 p.m. Let him watch the milk as it is poured, apparently pure, into the mixing vat Let

him then watch the scraping of the separators
(centrifugal machines) at the end of the day.
To strip off the tough, elastic layer from the
metal, it is necessary to use a strong scraper.
This layer, which is driven on to the wall of
the separator by the centrifugal force due to
about 6000 revolutions a minute, is made up of
hairs, dust, cobwebs, pieces of straw, particles
of cow-dung—scraps, in fact, of every sort
possible in a cowshed. These varieties of dirt
are bound in a matrix of mucus, epithelial
scales, and such other slimy matter as may
be separated from the milk. Experiment
has shown that milk bacteria are perceptibly
reduced in number, but not entirely eliminated, by the process of centrifugalisation,
and probably the germ population of the in-
spissated débris described is proportionally
greater than in corresponding volumes of milk.

But even if the germ-population of the
milk is not very seriously reduced, the milk
is made more limpid, and consequently more
palatable. At the very least, the consumer
does *not* want to consume either cow-dung
or cobwebs ; hairs *might* be, if they are not,
filtered out by the ordinary sieves ; epithelial
scales and minute amounts of mucus are
neither here nor there. But, for my own
part, ever since I first saw and realised the
amount of this lining deposit, which not in-

frequently is nearly a hard half-inch thick, I have never been able quite to *feel* that non-centrifugalised milk is as clean as centrifugalised milk. Partly this is, no doubt, a prejudice, or rather a revulsion, due to seeing facts out of relation to the whole they belonged to. For, in a drinkable quantity of milk, the few epithelial scales, broken hairs, straw particles, or particles of organic dirt, would not, for the moment, appreciably alter its physical qualities. But, as I have shown, germinal dirt affects the " keeping " qualities of the milk, and the germinal is not in fact separable from the non-germinal. The milk is heated before, and cooled after, separation ; and it is true that, with no further treatment, separated milk " keeps " longer than non-separated. Whether it be that the removal of the non-germinal dirt removes mechanically a large percentage of bacteria, or that the dirt removed reduces the nutrient quality of the medium, I am unable to say. Perhaps, independently of either alternative, the flavours of the milk are improved by the removal of foul organic substances that would normally form excellent material for bacterial putrefaction. One fact the " separation " demonstrates, namely, that the ordinary cowshed or dairy sieve (or filter) does *not* remove any but the major varieties of dust

particles. But there are many more efficient
sieves in the market. (Separation and centrifugalisation may be taken here as meaning
the same. The milk and cream can be, and
often are, re-mixed after separation.)

In thus painting, with a broad pencil, the
dirt conditions, I have omitted the aggrava-
tions due to ulcerated teats, inflamed udders,
pustular conditions, and the like. To realise
what these amount to, one must examine a
few large dairies. For curiosity, I have sometimes gone round a cowshed of a hundred cows
or more. The percentage of abraded teats
would astonish any but a practised milker
or inspector. This is easy to explain. To
begin with, the conditions of the milk cow
are largely pathological. The appropriation
of her by the human milker compels certain
modifications and adaptations. The ever-
renewed dragging at the teats leads to hyper-
trophy, congestion, and increased vascularity.
Normally, the teat is tender, easily abraded,
easily inflamed. If the cow is on pasture, she
may have the teats scratched or pricked by
thorns, whins, brambles, or the like. If she
is, as commonly in towns, entirely confined
to the cowshed, coarse bedding, bad floors,
or the innumerable accidents of movement,
may irritate or injure. Obviously, want of
protection exposes the teat to many injuries.

Twice or three times a day these injuries are aggravated by rough, mechanical handling. The gentlest human hand hardly matches the " toothless gums " of the calf. And the hand of the milker is, as a rule, far from gentle. I speak from observation of many scores of town and county dairies. At least half of the milkers, if not more, are men, who, in their ordinary labour, develop the normal " horny hand," and cannot divest themselves of it at the moment of milking. And the hands of the women-milkers are not softer and not often cleaner.

Then, in calving time, the puerperal cows occupy the same cowsheds as the non-puerperal. In such a time, the increase of organic putridity must be enormous. But the milk market is unaffected,—except for the increased quantity of milk.

One could add to these facts indefinitely. I mention only things visible in ordinary dairies. Then who shall enumerate the passing ailments of the milker ? Head colds, sore throats, ranging from evanescent redness to complicated diphtheria, inflamed fingers, inflamed eye-lids, conjunctivitis, acne, ringworm, eczemas in their varieties, and the large range of minor diseases that are more or less septic in their effects. Bronchitis and the like, I may leave alone.

When these commonplac. .acts are clearly grasped, and set coherently in the imagination, they teach one to estimate how much the "lime-washing in April and October" has to accomplish; how ridiculously futile are the efforts at enforcing cleanliness, when every movement means more dirt; how miserably on the outside of the disgusting facts are the provisions for lighting, ventilation, and cleansing. These provisions, however, are not without value; for they are forcing into prominence the minimal conditions of wholesome managements of cowsheds.

Turn now to the dirt incidental to the distribution of milk. The distribution of milk is as difficult a problem as the preparation of it before distribution. Our current methods are of the crudest. Recently the structure of the carts and of the cans has shown some regard to the cleanly handling of a delicate liquid; but there is yet a vast amount to improve. Then, consider for a moment the ordinary town milkshop. Exceptions, handsome exceptions, there are, doubtless; I speak of the ordinary shop. It is placed in a busy thoroughfare. It is every hour of the day frequented by the people of the locality. They come from every grade, and

in every variety of dress. The door opens
and shuts every five minutes—now to receive
supplies, now to serve an urchin. " A
penny'sworth o' skum milk," he says. " We
have no skim milk," replies the shop-maid.
" Weel, then, gie's sweet." He comes from
a poor home ; his hands, not long ago, have
been assisting at the cleansing of a street
gully ; but he takes the milk home in an
open jug, placing it, perhaps, on the ground
in order to have another turn at the gully.
As he left the shop a gust of wind blew in
some dust. The milk-vessels on the counter
were open to receive it. In some cases, it
is true, the vessels are covered ; in a few
cases, they are kept in a glass cupboard ;
but any milk-seller of experience will tell
you that milk shut off from the air is less
pleasant to drink. He is, of course, thinking
of raw milk, as it comes to him from the byre
—half-cool and but roughly sieved. Probably he is right. As milk absorbs odours
very readily, so it may part with them
sooner on exposure. It is certain that in
butter-making free exposure to the air during
the churning dissipates certain disagreeable
odours. Anyhow, a glass case would protect from dust without preventing aëration.

But to return to the shop's environment.
Once a day the cleaning cart comes round

Like as not, the ash-bucket is tilted into the
cart and pitched down just opposite the door.
The dust is naturally borne where its chance
of alighting on the milk is greatest.   Meanwhile, look further in.   That door goes, by
a short passage, to a living-room behind—a
kitchen, bedroom, scullery, and workroom
all in one.   That is the inviolable freeman's
house, which is his castle.   The short passage
is sometimes reduced to two doors, separated
by three or four feet.   That is " indirect " as
opposed to " direct " communication.   The
" short passage " is, in fact, a legal subterfuge
to evade the Dairies Order.   From and to
the shop the children run all day.   Perhaps
groceries are sold ;   perhaps only eggs and
butter ;   much more frequently, confections ;
rarely is the shop devoted exclusively to milk,
milk products, and accessories like eggs.
Then the shop goods must be dusted ;   they
must be arranged from time to time ;   they
may, in many shops, stand until the dust
covers them ;   and then every swing of skirt
or cloak or shawl, every current of air,
sets something more floating milkwards.
Perhaps, again, mangling and milk-selling go
together.   Perhaps the means of scalding
the plates and pails are inadequate.   To
describe every variety of combination legally
permitted is impossible.   What I have said

is enough to demonstrate that, if the dirt
of the cow-shed is enormous, the possible dirt
of the milk-shop is little less.

And if, to the inevitable dirt of the cleanest
town environment, one adds the dirt of
infrequently washed hands, uncut nails, shed
skin, fouled sleeves, and the innumerable
abominations of pent-up life in single rooms of
town houses, one cannot but stand amazed
at the capacity of the civilised palate to feed
on polluted supplies.   It is necessary to add
—clothes that go for months unwashed ;
beds unaired ; blankets washed once a year ;
adults and children that have never had a
bath of the whole body.   In places like these,
a surgeon would exercise the most stringent
care in his endeavour to secure asepsis, even
for a minor operation ; a major operation he
would not tackle.   But the same surgeon, if
bacteriology has not cured him of his milk,
often as not permits his kitchen staff to supply
his children with milk from the very shop
where he would not operate.

Here, then, is a serious problem.   The
hygienic solution is simple enough.   Let
milk-shops be constructed on the same lines
as an aseptic operating theatre ; let the
principles of the laboratory be applied to the
protection of the milk ; let the shops be

devoted exclusively to the sale of milk and
milk products ; let there be no communication with living-rooms ; let there be air ;
let there be light. To fit up a shop with
impervious walls, shelves, counters, etc., is
an affair of every day. To provide protecting cases for the milk, to separate old milk
from new, to reduce the need for manipula-
tion to a minimum—these are easy problems
hygienically, and, now and again, they are
solved. But for the most part they are
blocked by the " economic " incidents of the
vast trade in milk.

Did space allow, it would be profitable to
consider how the consequences of all these
pollutions can be, at least partially, averted,—
by mechanical cleaning, by complete sterilisation, by partial sterilisation (pasteurisation),
and other methods. Milk, too, is often the
means of spreading enteric fever, scarlet
fever, and diphtheria in large and sudden
epidemics. It is probably a leading cause in
the spread of tuberculosis. There are legal
means of countering these effects,—dairy
regulations, cleansing of persons, inspection,
construction of buildings, etc. But the hygienic difficulties are complicated by economic
difficulties ; for the milk trade is a very
great trade, and the need for milk induces

the consumer to take risks. But legislation
steadily grows more exacting ; opinion, more
informed ; organisation, better adjusted.   Yet
we are far off even from ideals immediately
possible.   But the " soured milk " treatment
continues to spread.   The needs of infants
and children more and more impress the
public mind.   The values of milk, butter, and
cheese are more appreciated in the dietaries.
Everything points to an enormous demand for
milk.   The day may come when, as a distinguished student of reform suggests, pure milk
may be " laid on " like water, gas, or elec-
tricity.   If that day should come, the present
dirty methods of producing milk will disappear like the polluted water supplies and
the unlit streets—only more rapidly.

CHAPTER XIII

THE HOUSE AS IMMEDIATE FAMILY ENVIRONMENT OR HOME

THE family is an incipient city.   The city
is an organisation of services to express, to
develop, and to protect the growth and

functions of the family. The rural cottage, the farm-house and its cot-houses, the estate mansion-house and its group of service houses, the village, the small town, the town, the great city, all, in their degrees, embody the services necessary to let father, mother and child grow to their full social functions. The needs of the family determine the evolution of the city. The limit of civilised subsistence in the city is the one-roomed house for the minimum family of father, mother, and infant. But, at the sacrifice of health, decency, and, therefore, morals, the limit is usually overstepped. The result is the slum and its population of de-civilised families. This is the primary problem of town-planning.

Consider the functions of the home. They are, primarily, to shelter parents and children. As to parents, the home must provide housing adequate to the occupation of the bread-winner ; it must provide means of storing and cooking food ; it must provide facilities for washing clothes and body, for clearing away waste, for maintaining cleanliness ; it must leave space for the occupations of leisure, for the treatment of disease, for the growth and education of families. As to children, the home must provide nursing, feeding, cleansing, education. All these the house must make possible ; for to be a home is the highest function of a house.   The home is the focus of social activities, the head-quarters of the functional social unit.   The home is the home of the family, and the family needs shelter, food, clothing, education, and medical care.

But the home is not alone the stone walls where our father and mother and brothers and sisters live.   Home is there only where a man will wish to turn when his day's work is done : it may be the shelter for wife or child ; it may be the birthplace of sister or brother ; or again, it may be the hermit's hut on the mountain-side, where solitude is the one companionship ; or yet again, it may be the open moorland, where freedom is and where " the wind blows on the heath."   And they that live in the ideal may be " citizens of the world " ; to them the whole earth is their domain, and one place like any other place fulfils the purpose of humanity.

How does the house of the town worker answer our description ? How shall this suite of mean rooms—undecorated, uncleaned, unaired, odorous, crowded, unhandsomely domestic, and dull—how shall this focus of broken interests, and starved ideals, and petty disappointments, and spiritless resignations —how shall this temple of broken gods be a home, a haven to run for in a storm, an altar to weep on in sorrow, a pillar of fire to guide him in the tangle of living ? How shall he enter into his chamber in silence for communion with holy things when he cannot get beyond the common noises of the day, the squalling of children not his own, the offence of cooking food, or the greater offence of spilled alcohol ?

Compare the rural worker and the town worker. The rural worker has his open door ; he can walk miles without meeting another like himself ; he has fields to roam in, hills to climb, trees to shade himself under, streams that croon to him when he is weary and guide his imagination when he is glad. Compared with the invasive dust and din of the town, his day is a perpetual Sabbath of cleanliness and quiet. But he, too, has his life of the slums ; no more than the town-dweller has he learned the uses of a house ; he oftener keeps it clean, because there is less dirt to invade it ; but he as often keeps his windows shut and sleeps in space too little for his dog. With all his advantages of open sky and clean air, the rural worker is not so far in front of the town artisan as the mere living in the country seems to indicate. Often, he is far behind. He suffers from damp houses, badly built, in bad situations. He has difficulty in keeping the soil clean, in removing refuse, in providing for the elementary decencies. All over, given equal physique, he is more vigorous; for he has freer access to the greater goods of light and air, and, which is equally important, he is less exhausted by the routine of his labour and the multitudinous attacks that the town life makes on the senses of eye and ear. He is slow in his actions, for he has to keep pace only with the seasons and the cows; not with cars, cabs, and trains.

Consider, too, the worker's wife. She is compelled to be industrious; she has the children for her daily burden. Usually, she makes the children's clothing; she keeps them constant in their school attendance; she assists them at lessons; she reports their illnesses; she trains their characters. I know of no better ethical teacher than a good artisan's wife. She is always in touch with reality. She has manners; she has intelligence; she has foresight; she has ambition. But often she runs under a heavy handicap. She interviews the factor when the drains are choked; she abuses him when he fails to repair them; she pays the rent, she pays the rates, she banks the wages in the friendly society. " I paid his society money for sixteen years, but he was aye ill and over-wrocht. I fell back wi' the instalments, and now I'll no' get a penny." She was the widow of a hard-worked riveter, who had given himself a sacrifice for children and wife, dying of overwork at forty, and leaving his wife to continue the battle.

How shall we relieve the pressure of this domestic drudgery ?

To begin with, there are the children. The problem of the children has been in part solved already. The older of them go to school ; they remain there for a fair proportion of the day ; they come home again, or remain for a time on the street, and on the whole they are not too much of a burden to the weary and heavy-laden mother. But the children of less than school age ? One is six months old, and demands constant nursing. Another is eighteen months or two years old, and demands constant supervision. A third is three and a half or four years old, and is just capable of getting constantly into mischief. There may be others, but we shall rest at three. To do full justice to the life of one infant would require more than all the mother's energies, and she has to divide herself among three. Nor that only ; she must prepare her husband's meals—at least three in the day. She may have a lodger, and she must prepare his meals — at least three in the day. She must feed the school children—three times a day. She must wash,

she must scrub, she must mend, she must
buy, she must cook, she must bake, she
must suckle the one baby and keep the other
moderately clean and the third moderately
safe, she must all day and most of the night
give of her soul and body to the needs of
others ; but one thing she must never do,
she must never fall out of temper, and she
must never feel tired. Is it a wonder if
now and again the brave heart begins to
weary, and the eyes to water, and the lips
to pale, and the limbs to tremble, and the
breath to come fitfully, and the stairs to
grow heavy, and the body to grow thin, and
the interests to grow narrow, and the desire
of life to run low, and the world to be too much
for her, and the very flesh at last to cry out
for rest—" Give us long rest or death, dark
death or dreamful ease " ? Is it any wonder
if she gives the biggest contribution to the
consumption death-total—she that cannot
venture into the air because she cannot carry
the baby, and rarely sees the sun ? Do we
need any more to explain why the friendly
societies are there ? why the doctor is kept
busy ? why infection multiplies ? and why
even a slum grows tolerable to its inmate ?
It is not that they prefer darkness, and bad
air, and perpetual labour ; it is that the life
they grow into is beyond their individual

strength. They must go under ; they do go under.

Take a walk with me down to Newhaven. This young woman has lost her husband. He was a young fellow of good character— capable, steady, reliable. One night, on his way home from his night-work on the railway, he dropped down ill. His companion ran to the nearest hospital ; he was taken there and, on examination, he was found to be suffering from severe bleeding of the lungs. He was kept until he had recovered sufficiently to be sent home. A week later he took a sudden bad turn and died. On hearing of his death, I called at the house. There I found some sympathetic neighbours, who had shown the young widow her duty. She was calm ; she belonged to good people ; she rested on human sympathy. She took me to the room where her husband lay, telling me how he had died. There, in a room as clean and tidy as if it were in a palace, lay the dead man, covered over with sheets of spotless white— the last sacrifice on the altar of personal devotion. The baby smiled and kept to its mother, and all was peace and quietness and brave character.

Later, I saw the young woman again ; but this time her dream had long gone by and she was once more the Newhaven fisherwoman—clean, powerful, foresighted, equal to the fate imposed upon her. It is with regret that one watches the covering over of that ancient and powerful people; the very houses are vanishing under our eyes: the individuality of race is invincible, but the individuals of it are becoming less and less numerous.

Surely it is not hopeless to think that something of the fine energy of these peoples of the sea-border might find a parallel in the streets farther inland; or must we, after all, accept the depressing conclusion that, as the freedom and risks of the sea made that great race of fishermen—strong, independent, competent, fatalistic—so the grinding monotony of the ordinary industrial life of the towns makes a race of feeble body, unsatisfied mind — hopeless, heedless, unstirred by any excess of " the will to live " ? One cannot think of this as a permanent consequence of industrialism, even if it be for the time inevitable. In a town of varied occupations, all types are to be found—from the dejection of the dirtiest slum-labourer to the buoyancy of the full-blooded carrier from the country. The continued infusion of fresh country blood is the salvation of the towns; and usually, though the incomers are deeply grieved at the town dust and dirt, they do, on the whole, maintain a higher standard of management in their houses than the older generations of town-dwellers. But even among the less vigorous of our people, the environment plays an enormous part; and I am satisfied that the energies of life can be organised to far greater purpose if only the fearful waste of a bad environment could be eliminated.

When this is thoroughly understood, some consequences grow clear. The school is a necessity; the hospital is a necessity; the industrial school is a necessity; the day-nursery is a necessity; the nursery-school is a necessity; everything that increases the energy of the home by reducing the friction to be overcome is, from the standpoint of social progress, a necessity. As things are, the home ceases to be a home because it is overweighted with the squalid and the unworthy. Remove these by better external organisation, and the home at once has a chance of rising into the most intimate of social clubs.

One morning, about five o'clock, it was my painful duty to visit a workman's house to inform his wife that he was dying in hospital. The door was opened by a child of five. She had risen from her temporary bed on the floor ; she had been suffering from measles. In the other bed lay the mother and four other children, arranged as the accidents of coverings would permit : the oldest child was, perhaps, twelve ; the youngest, a few weeks. Six people slept in the one room, and this is hardly to be called overcrowding compared with some cases I could give. This house, however, was the home of a respectable workman, who would have earned some 30s. or £2 a week steadily. Trouble had come upon him ; health failed ; the spirit had gone out of him ; poverty began to take possession ; then he died, and the mother with her five had to face the pitiless world. In cases like these, where shall we begin with a remedy ? And they are to be counted by the hundred. Yet this brave woman has faced the desert, and she has not fainted by the way. The oldest girl has gone to some occupation. The others go to school. The baby is in hospital. The mother will, by the help of one institution and another, climb up again into the circle of efficient citizens ; adversity has tried her and tempered her ; it has not subdued her. If one could help her by the impersonal service of some institution to nurse her weakest from time to time, she would gain in energy without losing in effort ; society would be a true providence, seeking no reward but the reward of renewed endeavour after new life.

Even overcrowding has its good side. The family of the working man is thrown so much together that the children instinctively cling to one another. Here, for instance, is a mother with five children. The oldest is about fourteen, the youngest is five months. One of them has German measles and a cough. Another has a sore throat. The mother is herself suffering from the bad weather. It is about ten in the morning. They have just risen—those of them that are able. The baby and the two patients are yet in bed with the mother. The father has gone early, but he will be home again in the evening. Squalor, do you say ? Unhappiness ? Not a bit of it ! The baby is eyeing us all placidly ; " she hath but wondered up at the white clouds." The three-year-old at the bed-foot is gazing with newly opened eyes at the intruders. The oldest boy, half-dressed, is kissing his hand and snapping his fingers to the baby. The oldest " girlie " is exploding every second with laughter at this little wondering wonder. Even the mother, anæmic, depressed, smiles with them. The house is not yet cleaned ; it may not be to-day ; it is not tidy ; the breakfast dishes are not cleared away ; a stocking is lying here, a petticoat there ; kitchen and bedroom are one and the same. Yet have we not here for the moment, could we but keep it, the very essence of the ideal family—the romance of innocence, fresh love untouched with worldliness, spontaneous service, self-sacrifice, the will to live, the joy of life ? In every family those moments come ; perhaps among the poor they are more frequent than among the comfortable, where personal service becomes often too conscious of itself and passes into sentiment ; but they come only to pass again, and the very problem we are seeking to understand is how to convert those sparks from heaven into the steady light of our everydays.

Now, further, as to this overcrowding. Let us analyse a little. What amount of space does a healthy adult need to breathe in ? To this no one answer is possible. But assume that we are thinking of a dwelling-house where a man may have to sit or move about for an average of three or four hours of an evening. To keep the carbonic acid of the fouled air down to 6 parts per 10,000, he will require about 3000 cubic feet of air per hour ; in three hours he will need 9000 cubic feet. That is, if the room is 10 feet wide, 10 feet long, and 10 feet high, the air in it must be completely changed three times every hour. Most working men's kitchens are rather larger than this; but furniture reduces the available space. We may assume a room of 1000 cubic feet as a fair standard.

But the man is rarely alone. There is his wife; there are the children; say, six persons in all. Often as not there is a stranger. Suppose we say that the room's average population will be, at a low figure, equivalent to five adults. As each adult requires 3000 cubic feet of air per hour, five will require 15,000 cubic feet. But we have omitted something very important. The house is lit with gas, and the gas burner consumes, say, five cubic feet of coal gas (mixed, I believe, with some so-called " water gas," or hydrogen and carbonic oxide) per hour. The gas pollutes the air as the human individual does. Each cubic foot of coal gas burnt per hour is, roughly, equivalent in polluting effect to half an adult; five cubic feet will be equivalent to two and a half adults, or, say, in round numbers, three adults. We thus have, in our 1000 cubic feet, eight adults, each requiring 3000 cubic feet of air per hour, that is, 24,000 cubic feet in all. Air costs absolutely nothing; it is absolutely essential to life; yet where are these eight adults (five of them alive and three of them simply a gas burner) to get it ? Not by the kitchen window, for it was shut as soon as the light went in and the blind went down ; not through the door, which is kept shut to keep the neighbours and the cats and other children and thieves out ; not by the parlour window, for that is open only once a week or so, for fear the rain might get in or the light spoil the carpet. If you stand up on a chair, after two hours of this " home life," you soon come down again, for the upper levels of the air are reeking with burnt gas and hot vapour. The baby falls asleep ; the mother says it is because he has been out so much, and perhaps he was out an hour in the morning. The school children grow hot in the cheeks and dull in attention. They gradually grow drowsy and go to bed. The father and mother soon follow—weary and yawning.

Next morning the room is colder ; the fire has gone out ; they have breathed some of the air for the hundredth time ; the father brushes himself up, gets out into the open air, lights his pipe, and by the time he reaches his work he is positively fresh. The mother never gets out all day, and never gets fresh. The children soon knock off the depression. But the baby gets the worst of it ; he must wait until he is taken out. The windows at last are opened, and there is a temporary return to nature and sanity.

So far I have spoken only of the functions of the house. Functionally, as we see, the two- or three-roomed house is really a one-roomed house. If this be the result with two rooms or more, what shall we say of the real one-roomed house ? Its condemnation was written in words of fire by Dr. J. Burn Russell of Glasgow. I have read no more terrible indictment of a social system. And it was written out of a wealth of detailed knowledge probably unsurpassed in the world.

The need of a good home is the driving power behind all the movements for the better Housing of the Working Classes and for the better Planning of Towns. This is not the place to discuss remedies. But one general danger I may emphasise.

There is a tendency to separate the Town Planning movement from the movement for improving individual houses. This tendency is natural, and the influences that create it are easily analysed. There is the Building interest, which looks for more possibilities of renewing its activity as soon as one area is built up. There is the Land interest, both owning and speculative, which naturally wants to sell or use land to the best financial purpose. There is the Architectural interest, which sees in every new scheme of an extended town fresh opportunities of artistic development. There is the Hygienic interest, which welcomes at all hands the spreading of the town over a wider area, if thereby the congestion of the centre is relieved. But, with the exception of the Hygienic interest, none of these pays special regard to the improving of individual houses. That is not for the moment their point of view. It is, however, the ultimately necessary point of view if the Town Planning movement is to result in improved dwellings. The value of the Garden City movement lies mainly in this, that it steadily combines the two standpoints—first, the provision of better houses for the individual dweller, and, second, the planning of the town to secure good æsthetic effects.

Between the two standpoints there is, or should be, no fundamental antagonism ; yet it is unquestionable that the tendency of the town-planner, as such, is to forget that the final test of town planning is not the production of artistic towns, but the improvement of individual housing. Professor Rudolph Eberstadt, of Berlin, who has given twenty years to the study of towns, maintains that the town - planning movement and the housing movement tend everywhere to conflict. On general grounds this is probable, and the proof of it is the city of Berlin itself. But the conflict is not necessary. If we watch the wave of building as it proceeds, decade by decade, we do, indeed, note that improvement of the margin goes hand in hand with deterioration of the centre ; but we also note that the new houses are individually rising to a higher standard, and that the demand for a higher standard continually asserts itself in the old houses too.

CHAPTER XIV

DISEASE AND DESTITUTION

DISEASE produces destitution ; destitution produces disease. Both propositions are true ; the evidence for both is overwhelming.

How does disease produce destitution ? Let us follow a case. Here is a workman earning £2 a week. He has a wife and five or six children, and keeps them in comfort. His wife develops tuberculosis of the lungs. She was, perhaps, infected early in youth, and now, overworked and underfed, rapidly becomes unfit for her duty. What is the husband to do ? He goes to his private doctor, who advises sanatorium treatment. But he finds sanatorium treatment beyond his means. He goes to a voluntary hospital in the locality, seeking admission for his wife ; but he finds either that they do not admit cases of the kind or that no beds are available. For a time, he keeps his wife at home, procuring the best treatment that his means afford. But, with no extra food, no fresh air, no constant medical direction, she grows no better and tends to grow worse. She may, at the same time, infect the children. The husband occupies the same room with her, possibly the same bed. He, too, may take the infection. At last he comes to the end of his resources. He cannot procure treatment for his wife and at the same time afford maintenance for his children. He has exhausted every source of voluntary assistance. He can no longer pay his doctor's bill. He applies to the Inspector of Poor. In Scotland, he would not be entitled to relief for his wife, because, by law, he is able-bodied, and no able-bodied person is entitled to relief. Legally, therefore, he cannot have his wife removed to the sick wards of the poorhouse ; but, if the Poor Inspector and the Parish Council are generous, they may, as they sometimes do, admit such a case to the poorhouse, and take the risk. The Public Health Authority is under legal obligation to take charge of the case; but, in many localities, the transfer from poor law to public health has hardly begun, and the poorhouse may be the most convenient destination, even if the Health Authority pay.

His wife is now provided for, and the household for a time thrives. But, driven by the cares of a sick consort and himself overworked, he gradually loses condition and ultimately shows signs of tuberculosis himself. The infection of a husband by a tubercular wife is said not to be common—statistically; but the infrequency of the occurrence does not help the individual case, and, whether infected by the wife or not, this man suffers from the disease. For a time he fights on; he asks for easier work; he has frequent periods off work, coming on his friendly society for sick pay. At last he is thrown out of his skilled occupation and falls into the ranks of unskilled labour. Here he finds that his children begin seriously to suffer. His wages are now inadequate for their full maintenance. The disease advances until he is entirely disabled. Then he goes through the same weary round as his wife, and ultimately joins her in the poorhouse, or in the Health Authority's hospital. The children are boarded out.

Pulmonary tuberculosis alone accounts for hundreds of cases like these. Any one that knows anything of the lives of an industrial town can add other illustrations from his own experience.

When tuberculosis of the lungs goes hand in hand with destitution, they move round in a vicious circle. The disease causes the destitution; the destitution aggravates the disease. This is above all true of tuberculosis; for an essential condition of recovery is the provision of excess nourishment. If you would have more evidence, go to the workhouse infirmaries of England, or the sick wards of the great Scottish poorhouses. There you will find cases in hundreds, not of phthisis alone, but of many other preventable diseases; and, if you track out their histories, you will, in many a case, find it difficult to determine whether the disease came first or the destitution came first. It is certain that they are bed-fellows now.

A poor person, suffering from non-infectious illness, has no claim on public funds unless he is destitute. He is, therefore, deterred by the conditions attached to the relief. It is, I think, accepted by all that destitution as a condition of medical service does, in a considerable degree, deter the really sick from invoking public assistance.

But this condition has a further consequence. It prevents the medical service of a destitution authority from ever becoming effectively preventive. Of the many preventable diseases already mentioned, some may, on occasion, lead straight to destitution and disablement. But the patient will not come to the Poor Law for treatment until no other treatment is to be had. A disease, therefore, that, in its acute state, might be easily cured and possibly prevented, tends by the delay to become chronic and incurable. This type of fact is accepted both by the Majority and the Minority of the recent Royal Commission on the Poor Laws. A deduction so obvious from premises so easily verifiable could scarcely be disputed. But if a medical service cannot be preventive, its maintenance must be in some proportion a waste of money. It is certainly true that masses of preventable disease are, at the present moment, untouched by any preventive medical service.

Look now at the Public Health service. It is grounded in the idea of prevention. Its administrative evolution has steadily followed preventive lines. It has shown in practice that masses of the infectious diseases are entirely preventable, that others are capable of control, that others are capable of amelioration. Everywhere, it goes on both improving the environment and providing for the individual.

But the movement has revealed another fact. It has shown that, between the infectious diseases proper and general diseases due to environment, there is no steady line of separation. The more the individual person is studied, the more his disease-conditions get allocated to environmental agencies. But this means that the concept of prevention must be extended. It cannot be any longer confined to the infectious diseases, great though that group is. Already the administrative organisations deal with the poisonings incident to certain trades, and do what preventive regulation can do to prevent their occurrence. But the preventive service can hardly stop at regulation. It will, in the course of events, pass on to the provision of treatment.

If this be so, the tendency to place disease on a footing independent of destitution will gather momentum. Every development of medical service within the last twenty years has followed preventive lines—notification of births, milk-depôts, health-visiting, medical inspection of schools. Any new developments, it is practically certain, must do the same. Fifty years of public health administration have educated the general mind in the advantages of early diagnosis by skilled people and early treatment in suitable institutions. The general opinion thus generated is not likely to stand still.

There are, I am aware, economic difficulties no less than administrative difficulties. But the economic difficulties will be at least in part surmounted by the next great step in the prevention of sickness, namely, obligatory Insurance of Workmen. To this let us now turn for a moment.

CHAPTER XV

INSURANCE METHODS OF PREVENTING SICKNESS

INSURANCE against sickness is not itself a preventive remedy, but it leads to prevention. This is the experience of every country that has organised compulsory insurance of workmen. Over twenty years ago, Germany established a system of compulsory insurance of wage-earners. The system did not begin with the open intention of preventing disease, but it has everywhere had that result. The best illustration is tuberculosis.

Recently, at an International Congress, Herr Bielefeldt, President of the Imperial Insurance Office, gave an account both of the insurance system and of the preventive methods developed under it. The benefits conferred by the insurance against sickness are chiefly these—first, sick benefit during disablement caused by a disease. Here the benefit runs for at least twenty-six weeks. In different localities, different amounts may be allowed, but the amount allowed must be at least half of the average earnings according to local usage. Second, assistance to the workman's family while he is treated in hospital. This money assistance amounts to half of the sick allowance. Third, money assistance for six weeks to women during confinement. The amount is equal to the sick pay. Fourth, in the event of death, an allowance to the parent of the deceased— this allowance amounting to twenty times the average daily earnings. So much for sickness insurance.

There are also certain allowances for

disablement extending beyond twenty-six weeks, and allowances for old age.

Here the wage-earner is under obligation to insure. The money so accumulated must be expended in his service. Insurance organisations have found that, in certain diseases, it is more profitable to treat early with a view to prevention than to wait till the patient is a permanent invalid. Tuberculosis is a striking example. In the early stages of insurance, all that was guaranteed was medical treatment and the necessary medicines. But the insurance associations were under obligation themselves to provide the medical attention and medicines. This led to a closer study of the problems of treatment. At first, no doubt, the associations tended to save money on the price of drugs. But, gradually, the conviction grew that the common interest of the association and its members lay in the rapid, efficacious and continuous provision of medical assistance. The number of doctors was increased. Specialists were engaged. Among others there were specialists for tuberculosis. It is to these considerations that the immense activity of the sickness insurance societies is due. Year by year they have expanded their scheme of treatment, always along the line of prevention. To-day it is possible for their members to have full advantage of the methods of modern medicine—the resources of bacteriology, of radiography, of hydro-therapeutics, electric treatment, massage, etc. In some cases, the associations allow to their members tonics in the form of milk, wine, various drugs, and mineral waters. In a serious case of tuberculosis, they offer gratuitously the service of nurses, or treatment at a watering-place, the open-air cure, and the like. There is also available treatment in a hospital or a clinic. Everywhere over Germany, as the result of experience, the sickness insurance associations have developed hospitals, clinics, and sanatoriums, all on preventive lines.

In whatever way, therefore, insurance against sickness may start, it necessarily ends in the development of preventive methods. The economic difficulties are thus partially solved. But many administrative difficulties remain. In Germany, when the system of insurance began, the public health movement, though it reckoned great names, was administratively not so fully developed as it is in Great Britain to-day. Doubtless, had the health organisations of town and county been fully organised, they would have been worked directly into the service. To some extent, indeed, they were. For,

in the leading German towns, hospitals for
the treatment both of infectious and of
non-infectious diseases are part of the municipal system. There are, of course, many
voluntary hospitals ; but, unlike our customs
in Britain, the treatment of general sickness
on the Continent has largely fallen to municipal hospitals. These institutions, therefore, are available as a working part of the
insurance system. To that extent, the
insurance societies have the advantage of
hospitals under public management.

In Britain, the course of administrative
evolution has been somewhat different. It
is only now, but with the advantage of continental experience, that insurance against
sickness is to be instituted. It proceeds
frankly from the beginning on preventive
lines. It will cover a large part of the field
of sickness and disablement. It therefore
necessarily takes with it the health authorities
everywhere established in England, Scotland,
and Ireland. These authorities, directly or
indirectly, will therefore have their bounds
enormously widened. They will be no longer
authorities merely for securing the sanitation
of the environment and the prevention of
infectious diseases. They will be animated
by a broader outlook They will scan the
whole environment as it is in relation to the

individual. They will push their analysis of the causes of disease until every producer of disablement is revealed, whether the disablement come from infection, or from poisoning, or from the dust diseases, or any other of the occupational diseases. The line between public health and individual health, always merely provisional, will at last disappear. The individual will no longer be in abstract antagonism to the community he lives in ; he will, even by his cash nexus, find himself an organic unit of the greater organisation.

And so a system of individual insurance reveals new social relationships. The system shows itself as, after all, only a specialisation of the public health movement. That movement began with an inspection of the grosser defects of the environment ; it ends with a minute scrutiny of the individual. Yet the line of evolution is perfectly continuous. At no stage can it be said, here is a definite end. There can be no end until the individual, in his passionate desire for health, finds that the common health service is the only instrument that can achieve his individual aims.

It was this high purpose that created the scheme of National Health Insurance presented to the House of Commons by Mr. Lloyd

George, Chancellor of the Exchequer, on the
4th of May 1911, a red-letter day in the history of industrial democracy. The scheme
is, perhaps, the most comprehensive scheme
of Health Service that has yet emerged in
any civilisation. It has in it the beginnings
of a vast revolution in medical organisation.
It concerns the daily lives of some fifteen
millions of people. It brings the enormous
individual energies of the great Friendly
Societies into relation with the social energies
of the public organisations. It is a new correlation of social forces to prevent disease and
to establish health. And, politically, it has
caught the imagination of all sections of
society It has stilled the criticism of the
political partisan. It has evoked the cool
consideration of the expert. It has persuaded
the mind of the man of business. It has
opened before the eye of the worker new ways
in the wilderness of living. It has devised
new services for the health authorities. It
provides them with resources for the extension
of their beneficent activities. The Chancellor's exposition of his scheme showed that the
measure was a great one. The impression is
but deepened by the detailed study of the
Bill.

The State arranges for the collection of the
funds. By Mr. Lloyd George's original pro-

posals a workman would contribute 4d. a week, a workwoman 3d. a week, the employer 3d. a week.   The State would contribute two-ninths of the benefit in the case of men and one-fourth in the case of women.   Certain classes of worker are excluded.   But certain classes may be admitted as voluntary contributors.

The funds are distributed by the State through two channels—first, the Friendly Societies; second, a special organisation named the "Local Health Committee."   The Friendly Societies must be approved by the State, and must undertake to provide for their members certain minimum benefits.   For those not in Friendly Societies, the State distributes the collected money through a Local Health Committee, representing four main interests— the local authorities for public health, the Friendly Societies, the insured persons not in Friendly Societies, and the State itself.   This Committee is the principal new creation of the Bill.

What form shall the distributed money take ?   Look first at the minimum benefits made possible by the contributions of workman, employer, and State.   For all those insured in Friendly Societies, there must be the following : The insured person will receive medical attendance throughout life.

The allowance in sickness according to the original Bill would be at the rate of 10s. a week for men and 7s. 6d. a week for women for thirteen weeks from the fourth day of sickness, and 5s. for the next thirteen weeks. For the remainder of sickness, however long it lasts, the insured person would receive 5s. a week. A provision of immense value is the provision for maternity benefit, to be received if the mother is either herself insured, or is the wife of an insured person. As the Old Age Pension system already in force provides for persons over seventy, the benefits under the present scheme cease at that age.

Out of the whole contributions a proportion per person insured must be set aside for a Sanatorium Fund. This fund will be controlled by the Local Health Committee. It will be used for the provision and management of sanatoria of all kinds—sanatoria for tuberculosis being at the moment the most prominent. But other diseases may also be provided for. Further, a substantial vote would enable local authorities and others to provide sanatoria and other institutions for the treatment of tuberculosis and such other diseases as the Local Government Board may appoint, this sum being distributed by the Local Government Board, which, as the central authority for health, controls the whole health policy of the local authorities.

There is another major provision. If, in any locality, there is any excess of sickness among the insured, the Local Health Committee or a Friendly Society may demand an inquiry by the State Department concerned— the Home Office, for instance, or the Local Government Board. If the excess of sickness can be shown to be due to the conditions or nature of the employment, or to bad housing, or to insanitary conditions in any locality, or to defective or contaminated water-supply, or to the neglect on the part of any person or authority to observe or enforce the provisions of any Act relating to the health of the workers in factories, workshops, mines, quarries, or other industries, or relating to public health, or the housing of the working classes, or any regulations made under any such Act, or to observe or enforce any public health precautions,—then the various persons or bodies concerned may have to make good the difference of expense due to the excess of sickness so caused. These provisions are of immense range, and place the prevention of disease on the bed-rock of personal money interest.

The Bill also contains a scheme for insurance against unemployment. But this concerns health only indirectly, and may here be disregarded.

The details for the realisation of these great ends occupy in the original Bill nearly eighty large pages of foolscap.   The experience of other countries has been taken as a guide, not as a model.   The special conditions of British society have led to the great proportional part played by voluntary organisations.   And the contributing persons control the destination of their contributions.   But the official health authorities receive not only new powers, but new stimulus to use them.   As time goes on, the movement towards prevention will steadily increase in volume.   The health of the person and the health of the community will be once more revealed as but two phases of a single problem.

And this leads to our last chapter, where all the threads are woven into a flowing pattern, which is the progressive synthesis of prevention and cure.

CHAPTER XVI

THE EVOLUTION OF THE HEALTH MOVEMENT

DR. J. BURN RUSSELL struck a high ethical note in his *Evolution of the Function of Public Health Administration.*

He spoke not as an administrator only. He was a stern pleader for social righteousness. The burden of his twenty-six years of administration was—" Comfort ye, comfort ye my people." How much Scotland and the world owe to his personal devotion none can conjecture except those that knew him. But the city of Glasgow published a Memorial Volume of his writings. And there the record of a great and patient administrator can be read. He could clothe statistical dry bones with the flesh and blood of an informed social doctrine. His diagrams have passed into the text-books ; his intensive studies of housing are classics in their kind ; but the science of them was informed by a singular righteousness and potency of conviction.

The story his writings tell is a marvellous one. It reveals the progress of a community more convincingly than any mere history of institutions. It lays bare the nerve of social health, the minimum conditions of individual growth, the contrast between the listless neglect of fifty years ago and the skilled services of to-day. Surely the Service of Man owns no higher, no more honourable minister than him whose mission it is to cleanse, to purify, to sweeten the bright air, to shine the light into dark places, to fill with the joy of living the highways and byways, the alleys and the lanes, the courts and the wynds and the reeking cloisters of the social under-world. For in that dim land the primary ritual of nature has passed from the memory ; misery and filth clog the spontaneity of life and overload the will ; there is nothing but torpor and hunger and the melancholy vices of personal degeneracy.

Fifty years ago, Glasgow stood first among the cities of the kingdom for wretchedness, for filth, for the multifarious hordes of disease that follow them. But the fifty years saw the birth of a new movement, which is now sweeping round the world. In every great city the same problems have to be faced ; but the science of administration has gone steadily forward. Glasgow is but a type. How she shook herself free from the nightmare of typhus and all it meant ; how, through panic and error, she passed from one bad method to another less bad, and how at last, like all city organisations, she came to follow a policy designed and defined by a genuine social insight, form one of the finest illustrations of the transit from a vaguely felt social need to the scientific elaboration of an administrative system.

What one city in a hundred years of her history shows, every city in the world shows in its own degree and kind. For the movement towards health is world-wide. And it is not limited to the cities alone. There are the rural areas, more thinly peopled, it is true, but feeling their needs as warmly and developing their systems of administration as scientifically.

It was in 1889 that the great departure in rural administration took place in Scotland. It was then that the Parish as an administrative unit for public health was superseded by the County Council and the District Committees. For twenty years, the Public Health Acts in the counties had lain quietly on the parochial tables,—Acts that, in many of their provisions, were far in advance of the general opinions of their day. But I remember well how, as young medical officers of health, we were stirred by the new movement towards better social organisation. The field was wide. There were no guides to help us in our duty. Some of us had had experience in the towns ; some of us had to invent our experience in the counties. The irresponsible studies of the University had here to meet the hard necessities of administration in a world where individual houses were separated by miles, where the farms were incipient communities, where villages presented the problems of budding cities without the city resources, where, in a word, the whole common organisation was difficult to discover and more difficult to make effective. It was then that one felt how little the laws can do until the common heart is moving. But it did not take long to unlock the feelings of men in the counties. They were only waiting for a lead. The newly created county medical officers became the points of contact between the world of scientific ideas and the world of social needs. The hygienic conscience was awakening.

What was the material we had to work upon ? The whole range of rural life in farm, in village, and in small town. The farm is a simple social unit, which, on the whole, understands well the hygiene of animals, not so well the hygiene of men. Pigs must pay ; men are free. Pigs for pigs, therefore, are often better off than men for men. It is not one or an occasional farm, but many, I have seen, where absolutely the animals had more space, more air, altogether a healthier home, than the men that tended them.

It is natural ; for, unlike animals, men are held fit to house themselves. And, on the other side, the plain dispositions of farm life are not so easily offended ; a daily familiarity with dirt lets the sense for handsomeness drop, and nothing more astonishes a cowherd than to indicate how much cleaner his cowshed might be, or a long-lived crofter how much better aired his stables might be. If, thus, with animals, where good hygiene is so much in hard cash, the attention is not all it should be, how much worse is it with human beings, whose health is a secondary thing to their passing and seasonal efficiency It was the work of the medical officer to disturb this quiescence, to place the ideal higher, to generate a social sensitiveness that should regard filth as an indecency, defective ventilation as a breach of fashion, and more sleeping space as, at least, a legitimate ambition. In a lower middle-class house with what certainty may you find " oils " in the dining-room, engravings or etchings in the drawing-room, and not for worlds an ornamental tea-table in the breakfast parlour ! The poor man's ménage is less elaborate ; but there is much in it that he knows not how to use, or that he has caught a bad fashion of using. At least, he may be taught that windows should always open ; that chimneys should never be closed ; that if the kitchen is warmer in the winter, his spare room is fresher to feed in for the summer ; and that in illness " under the bed " is not a good place for odds and ends, least of all for use as a wardrobe. These defects of living the medical officer of health could bring to a clear consciousness ; he could initiate a " fashion " of healthiness ; and thus he could, as it were, sensitise the major decencies.

In our smaller villages the material was not much different. For what are our villages ? Here is one stuck down, a few houses at the meeting-point of two roads. The inhabitants are labouring people, farm hands, and the like ; shopkeepers, to supply the mixed group with food ; a carpenter's shop, a smithy, and not infrequently a common lodging-house. Sixty years or more ago, the mail coach passed this way ; that accounts for the inn, which now supplies alcohol to the group. The horses rested or changed there. By and by, another house got stuck down near the inn ; yet later the gregarious instinct, and perhaps the cheapness of useless land, produced another and another ; till now you see it—inn, schoolhouse, church, and village congregation. The houses are not ungainly; the walls are kept white, the windows black-bordered, the doorsteps clean; but what of sanitation? What of the water, for instance? There is the original well, enough for one, enough for two, for three; but too little for the group of families now constituting a community. New wells must be made; they are made. But in this haphazard, unguided growth, the assumptions of heedless farm life are slowly causing degeneration in the incipient town. For refuse accumulates; drains are not made; pigsties are not cleaned; ash-heaps are not changed; and the houses become unhealthy, damp, hardly habitable. And, a worse result, the wells are defiled. In our pastoral and agricultural counties this is the history of village on village. It is much to abate the major nuisances; it is more to teach their future avoidance; it is most, and most to aim at, to generate, in the affairs of health, the social feeling that keeps the walls white and the doorsteps clean. And this, it seems to me, was not beyond the scope of a medical officer's legitimate efforts.

What methods were devised to stir up the rural mind, I need not indicate; but to-day there is not a district of these com-

munities that has not better water, better
houses, better drainage, better hospital accommodation, than twenty years ago.   The
organisation of public health in Scotland has
everywhere advanced with an ever-increasing
acceleration.   To   those   that   knew   the
counties and some towns twenty years ago
and that know them now, the total difference
is barely credible.   Perhaps to the men
engaged in effecting the evolution, the progress has not always been the thing most
visible ;   but the progress has been vast.
Health authorities have become a reality.
Even the economic value of health has
become an impelling force.   District Committees, Burgh Councils, and County Councils
spend much time, energy, and money in giving
concrete form to the prescriptions of the
public health laws.   And these changes
followed on two main changes,—the areas
mere made large enough to let administration
become effective, and medical officers were
appointed to prevent disease.

But these are only local manifestations of
the Public Health movement.   In England,
it started consciously in the early years of the
nineteenth century, when Edwin Chadwick
was still young.   Chadwick's father, it is
worth mentioning, had seen Napoleon drilling
troops in the Champ de Mars, and it is not

far-fetched to believe that the younger Chadwick inherited some elements of the Revolution spirit. Anyhow, Chadwick is the great name in several beginnings, and certainly in the beginning of the modern Public Health movement.

His " Report on the Sanitary Condition of the Labouring Classes of Great Britain " was the result of Lord John Russell's commission in 1839, and remains to this day a classic in its kind. ·There is hardly a subject of interest to modern society that, at some stage, he did not handle and illuminate. The value of life, life as a commercial problem, life in prisons, days of sickness among the masses, dietaries, registration of births, marriages, and deaths, taxes on knowledge, the economics of intemperance, education, the physiological and psychological limits of mental labour, the half-time system, physical training for trade unionists, the construction of schools, pensions to school teachers, cheap railways, employers' liabilities, sewerage, cremation, over-crowding, ventilation, unhealthy trades, epidemics, war, poor-law, police, and the multitude of phenomena indicated by them,—these were the occupation of Chadwick's immense and unremitting energy. The organisations that flowed from the revolution achieved by the political

reform of 1832—reforms largely inspired and
guided by men like Chadwick and James Mill
and George Grote—gave scope for the development of a public health service in towns.   If
we had time, we might trace step by step
from these great initiations the modern
growth in local government, the organisation
of rural and village life, the vast expansions
of public health activities in county and
town.

Curiously, the Assistant, that is the active,
Secretary of the first Board of Health, which
Chadwick was the means of establishing, was
Alexander Bain, psychologist, afterwards
Professor of English and Logic and, later,
Lord Rector in the University of Aberdeen.
Chadwick was a friend of Bentham, and had
acted as his secretary.   He was an ardent
Benthamite.   These names are always
associated with the two Mills and George
Grote.   Not one of them was a medical man,
although Bain had studied in some of the
medical classes ; yet out of the social movements in which they were, in one degree or
another, leaders, grew the movement towards
Public Health.   It is not often that we can
associate a great movement so definitely
with the initiative of individual men ; but,
without straining the facts, we may really
regard the Public Health movement as a

specific application of Benthamite principles
to the improvement of society.

In the marvellously specialised organisation of our present-day health authorities,
with their skilled medical officers, medical
inspectors of schools, health visitors, nurses,
nuisance inspectors, fever hospitals, their
drainage districts, their water districts, their
housing, and their whole machinery for
administration of elaborate Public Health
Acts, it is difficult to discover any trace of
the social philosophy from which they have
all taken their immediate inspiration. But,
whatever be the particular origin, the Public
Health movement in Britain is one of the
finest examples of social growth known to us.
It is the name for a vast organisation that
has grown out of definite social needs ; it has
a perfectly defined objective ; it has methods
that can be analysed down to detail ; it is
steadily showing itself in new differentiations
and integrations. There is no section of society
unaffected by the movement; there is no section
that can disregard it ; there is no meanness of
finance that can escape it ; there is no inertia
that it will not ultimately overcome. Over
and over again, we see the bitter lesson driven
home on the reactionary mind ; over and
over again, the densest imagination must
waken up to a local need that disease, dis-

ablement, and death have revealed ; over and over again, the unhealthy locality, the unhealthy house, the death-dealing industry, and other innumerable varieties of insanitation have vanished under the tide of hygienic ideas.

If we turn from history, and look directly at the movement of the moment, we can detect at least one steady drift,—the drift from curative medicine to preventive medicine. The expert of the movement is the Medical Officer of Health. The evolution of this term would itself be an interesting study. Probably its first legal embodiment is to be found in the Public Health (Scotland) Act, 1897, where " Medical Officer of Health " is among the definitions. The phrase is now so common that over all England and Scotland it has shrunk to three capitals—M.O.H. That it should be only a few years old indicates the velocity of the movement. The term " Officer of Health " is an old one, and is not peculiar to England. Possibly also, " Medical Officer of Health " is older than I imagine ; but certainly it is only within the last twenty years that it has passed into social currency. The phrase is a crystallisation of the Public Health movement. It is " health " the movement aims at,—the establishing of every individual in his physiological normal. It is by " medicine " that this aim should be achieved,—the practical science of cure for the sick individual and prevention for him and his social group. And it is through an " officer " that the aim and the method come into synthesis,—the officer presupposing the organisation that determines his functions. The phrase, " Medical Officer of Health," therefore, is the embodiment of a new synthetic idea, which, on analysis, is no other than the transformation of cure into prevention, or rather the absorption of cure as a factor in prevention. The " doctor of medicine " thus reverts to his true place among other " doctors." He ceases to be the " leech " of old days, and becomes once more the teacher of health, the expounder of remedies. But the remedies are no longer applied to individuals alone ; they include the whole sweep of the environment as it affects the individual, and the individual as he is to be fitted to make his environment.

At first, naturally, the unspeakable abominations of the environment drew the fire of the Public Health services, and continue to draw it. But the effect has been, to some extent, a false abstraction. In elevating the environment, the Medical Officer of Health has tended to forget the individual organism. This he has left largely to his correlative, the " general practitioner." The Medical Officer tends to think of an abstract environment adapted to an average organism. He has developed great tables of birth-rates, of death-rates, and of disease-rates. He speculates on their rise and fall, as the stock-broker speculates on 'change, and he not infrequently forgets that his curves of averages, real though they be for their purpose, are only the symbol of actualities, not the actualities themselves. The more intensive has been his study of the environment and the more intense his efforts to improve it, the more he has tended to become dissociated from the care of the individual organism and absorbed in the preparation of abstract environments. Yet, ever and again, hour by hour, week by week, year by year, he is violently brought back to the needs of the individual. However much he may devote himself to the perfecting of water-supplies, the sites of new houses, the clearance of slum areas, the teaching of hygienic physiology, he can never get far away from the infected individual, who needs his definite assistance, and who, by his disease, reflects new light on the imperfections of the environment.

Meanwhile, however, other differentiations have been in progress. The medical inspection of school children has become a reality in England and in Scotland. The immediate point of departure for this new specialisation of duties was the Royal Commission on Physical Training (Scotland), whose report appeared in 1903. Few movements have developed so rapidly. New organisations have been created, or new developments of old organisations have been made. New officers have been appointed. In England, there are in the School Medical Service now approximately 1000 medical men, 73 medical women, and some 800 nurses. Large sums of money have been voted. Endless disputes have arisen. But the primary objective of the new specialisation is coming nearer and nearer, namely, the direct personal examination of the school child. It is no longer the environment; it is at last the individual. And it is not the individual alone, but the individual as he, by his defects and diseases, reveals all the relations he bears to the environment. Curative medicine and preventive medicine have come to a fresh synthesis in the medical inspection of the school child. The skill of the physician and the science of the Medical Officer of Health unite in the Medical Inspector of Schools.

And the Public Health movement cannot stop there ; for the school child, on his coming to school, brings with him the long history of his nurture and, on his leaving school, will bear with him into life the bias of his education. It follows that medical inspection of the school child must look backward into infancy and forward into adolescence and maturity. At every step the Medical Inspector watches the interaction of the individual and the environment, anxiously jealous that the environment shall meet the highest needs of the individual, and that the individual shall be strengthened to respond to the highest purposes of the environment.

There is now to follow a further specialisation of all the medical services   This will come as the result of the National Insurance for the prevention of sickness. Individual health and common health are at last seen to be one and the same.   What re-organisation of administrative functions this third new departure may involve, no one can foresee. The last twenty years cover a record of great changes ; but these are nothing to what the next twenty years will bring.   Let us, however, for a moment shift the point of view. It is natural, in these rapidly appearing developments, to look for fundamental principles.   They are not easy to put into words. Perhaps, the postulates of the Public Health movement, the movement towards individual

health, individual efficiency, are something
like these :—

The movement has its root in the ethical
effort after a richer, cleaner, intenser life in
a highly organised society. Society or the
social group is itself essentially organic. But
the social organism is an organism loosely
knit. It is capable of easy and rapid modification. When the modification is the expression of a real social need, it will survive ;
it will generate for itself the necessary administrative form. Disease, as we have seen
at the beginning, is a name for certain mal-
adaptations of the social organism or of the
organic units that compose it. These diseases, as has been abundantly shown, are in
greater and lesser degrees preventable. Their
prevention promotes social evolution. But
their prevention needs definitely organised
agencies. These are the administrative
bodies,—County Councils, Town Councils,
District Councils, Parish Councils, School
Boards, Imperial Government Boards, International Executive Committees. Through
these it is possible to control disease-producing
conditions, to prevent the onset of disease in
the individual, to permit society as a whole
and its individual citizens to benefit by all
the preventive methods from time to time
discovered or invented. Natural selection

may thus be definitely aided by artificial selection. Constitutional inheritance of disease may be, in some degree, compensated by more efficient social environment. By the continued modification of the social organism and its flowing environment, it is possible to further the production of better citizens,— more energetic, more alert, more versatile, more individuated.

The majority of the diseases that afflict the human body do not come from the body itself ; they come in the conflict between the human body and its environment. The environment includes all the organisms and conditions that operate as causes of death. These have been fully illustrated. Infectious disease, now a conflict between a higher organism and a lower, may be converted into a friendly co-operative life. The fatal and disabling trades may all have their fatality and disabling power reduced. The food environment is capable of indefinite improvement. And so on, through all the relations of men to each other and of all to the physical conditions of life. In its first stage, public health is the application of scientific ideas to the extirpation of environmental disease. In its second stage, it is the application of scientific ideas to the production of personal immunity. Everywhere, it is the synthesis of prevention and cure.   It is an organised effort of the collective social energy to heighten the physiological normal of civilised living beings.

And so the circle is completed.   The healthy individual man with whom we began needs a healthy community in order that he may maintain his physiological normals at their highest efficiency.

To these propositions many objections may be made.   Of these objections, I name two,— first, the charge that the Public Health movement exalts the environment at the expense of the individual heredity ;   second, that thus it evolves into a systematic method of reducing the pressure of life and thereby preserving the unfit.

As to heredity, the charge sits lightly upon us.   Any one that reads what has here been written must allow that the obstructions to healthy development are a vast and confused mass.   Until this gross environment is disentangled, split up, and reduced to its least potential, no one can know what the human organism can do.   If you give children more light, more air, more food, they will grow into healthier, stronger, more resistant adults than if you keep them in the dark, poison their air, and restrict their food.   To any one

that doubts this, I merely say : Try the
experiment of transplanting an infant from a
slum to a hospital. To go from the lightless,
airless, foodless home to the well-lit, well-
aired, well-provided hospital, is to go from
physiological poverty to physiological wealth.
Among the middle classes one never fails to
note the change from pinching to prosperity.
The thin, pale man with restless eye, anxious,
always thinking backwards, alters into the
rosy-cheeked, full-bodied citizen, with head
erect and a smile for all comers. In the less
favoured proletariat, the change is no less
striking. After a few weeks of light and air
and regular food, the human weakling sprouts
out and grows both in muscle and in nerve,
both in energy and in co-ordination, both in
body and in mind. It is not that new
faculties are created ; it is that old faculties
cease to be clogged up. And the sole change
has been a change in environment.

Until, therefore, the environment is first
made healthy, the question of physiological
inheritance does not concern the health
movement. It is an absurd waste to evolve
by natural selection an inheritable " fitness "
against an environment that can itself be
swept out of existence. In this country we
do not build houses in the tree-tops to escape
the wolves ; there *are* no wolves! Neither

do we kill thousands in order to evolve a
type fitted by heredity to resist plague ; we
simply keep plague out !

But a more fundamental answer may be
made.

It is our duty to prevent death. Out of
the effort to keep alive those that would
die of preventable diseases, the vast Health
Service has grown. Of what diseases *do*
we die ? Of what diseases *must* we die ?
These it is our duty to answer. Until the
secret of physical persistence is revealed, it
is ours to reduce the agencies of death to
those few that men must face and accept ;
to create, if it but be possible, new channels
for human energy, that the waste of living
may fall to its least and the wealth of living
—in breadth, in depth, in intensity—may
increase to the uttermost. Our service
meets heroic obligations. In despair, it is
not desperate. As the physician never
abandons the bedside until the breath ceases
and the pulse fades into rest and the limbs
lie without will and the eyes change their
lustre and there is no more man, so the
service of health watches the birth, the
adolescence, the full tide, and the ebb of
the social life. Never at any period is the
task abated. From the simplicities of the
primitive life on the hills, in the woods, in

the fields, along the rivers, and by the sea-
shore, to the infinite involutions of life in
the cities,—in the dust, in the noise, in the
dark,—our service is unremitting day and
night; it has its orders to administer, its
care to offer, its word for consolation. And
as men grow more from living to thinking,
as labour grows into knowledge, as the
nerves begin to dominate the muscles, and
as education, the arts, the sciences, the
crafts, catch the imagination of men and
intensify their interest for the invisible and
immaterial, the Health Service must grow
in subtlety to meet the keener diseases of
civilisation.

And, if it is given to any of us to watch
the decline and fall of any people, when trade
passes and hunger enters and famine glides
hither and thither telling who are the con-
demned, our service has yet its duty,—we
must be the last to go. If the phœnix may
not rise, we must yet prepare the funeral
pile and watch the flames die down.

So, through all the stages of the growth
of men in societies, the Health Service may
never be wanting. It is the form the Service
of Man takes equally in the day of his strength
and in the last phases of his decrepitude.

NOTE ON BOOKS

FOR a general conception of health, the reader may study one of the many elementary physiological handbooks, *e.g.*, Sir Michael Foster's *Primer of Physiology*, or Foster and Shore's *Physiology for Beginners* (both Macmillan & Co.). For death-rates, disease-rates, figures about epidemics, occupational diseases, etc., he may study the statistical section of any good manual or textbook of Public Health, *e.g.*, Whitelegge's *Hygiene and Public Health* (Cassell & Co.), or Lewis and Balfour's *Public Health and Preventive Medicine* (Green & Sons, Edinburgh), or Notter and Firth's *Theory and Practice of Hygiene* (J. & A. Churchill). These are all technical books, but contain much general information. For special details, Newsholme's *Vital Statistics* (Swan Sonnenschein), which is a standard handbook, may be consulted. On the problems of immunity, the most comprehensive book is Metchnikoff's *Immunity in Infective Disease*, translated by Binnie (Cambridge University Press).

Metchnikoff's book on *The Nature of Man*, translated with introduction by Dr. Chalmers Mitchell, F.R.S., and his small book on *The New Hygiene*, with preface by Sir E. Ray Lankester, contain much that is of immense importance for the study of diet and disease regarded from the higher standpoint of evolutional efficiency. Here is found the scientific basis of the " soured milk " treatment. As to diet, two of the most important works are Professor Chittenden's *Physiological Economy in Nutrition* and *The Nutrition of Man* (Heinemann). There are many good recent works on diet, *e.g.*, Dr. Chalmers Watson's *Food and Dieting*, Dr. Robert Hutchison's *Food and Dietetics* (Edward Arnold), Dr. Burney Yeo's *Food in Health and Disease* (Cassell & Co.). Books on vegetarian and special diets are without number. For food as a factor in the evolution of races, see Dr. Marion I. Newbigin's *Modern Geography* (Home University Library).

On general questions, the following will be found eminently interesting: *Hygiene of Nerves and Mind in Health and Disease*, by Dr. August Forel, translated by Aikins (John Murray) ; Dr. Clouston's *Hygiene of the Mind* ; also his *Unsoundness of Mind* (Methuen) ; Dr. Arthur Newsholme's *Prevention of Tuberculosis* (Methuen), *L'Hygiène moderne*, by Dr. J. Héricourt (Ernest Flammarion, Paris) ; *Manual of Natural Therapy*, by Dr. T. D. Luke (Wright & Sons, Bristol). *The Therapeutics of the Circulation* (Murray), by Sir Lauder Brunton, though technical, is well adapted for general study. Professor Arthur Thomson's *Heredity* (Murray) gives a perfect orientation on every question concerning diathesis, inheritance of disease, Weismannism, Mendelism, etc. Such a work makes an admirable biological discipline preliminary to the study of the whole field of disease. Other works are mentioned in the text.

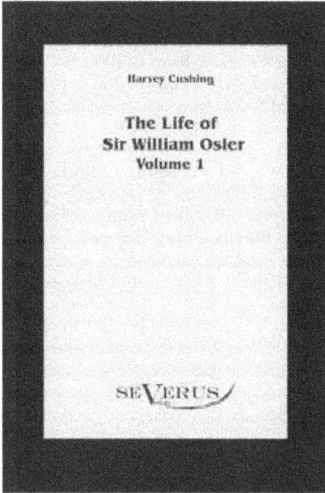

Harvey Cushing
The Life of Sir William Osler

Volume 1
SEVERUS 2010 / 700 Seiten / 39,50 Euro
ISBN 978-3-942382-26-7

Volume 2
SEVERUS 2010 / 696 Seiten / 39,50 Euro
ISBN 978-3-942382-30-4

William Osler (1849-1919) is widely regarded as one of the most influential physicians of the late 19th and early 20th century and a key figure in the history of medicine. Besides his research activities and his dedicated scientific work, Osler's greatest contribution to the medical world has been the system of residency which he developed at the Johns Hopkins Hospital in Baltimore, thus introducing a new and deeply humanistic approach to the strictly scientific realm of traditional medicine.

Harvey Cushing (1869-1939), a former student and close friend of Osler's and a pioneer of neurosurgery, has himself become an icon of modern medicine. He was one of the first physicians to use x-rays for diagnosing brain tumours, he developed revolutionary methods of blood pressure measurement, and he discovered Cushing's syndrome, the first autoimmune disease identified in a human being.
This monumental biography earned him the Pulitzer Prize in 1926.

Kerschensteiner, Georg Theorie der Bildung * Klein, Wilhelm Geschichte der Griechischen Kunst - Erster Band: Die Griechische Kunst bis Myron * Krömeke, Franz Friedrich Wilhelm Sertürner - Entdecker des Morphiums * Külz, Ludwig Tropenarzt im afrikanischen Busch * Leimbach, Karl Alexander Untersuchungen über die verschiedenen Moralsysteme * Liliencron, Rochus von / Müllenhoff, Karl Zur Runenlehre. Zwei Abhandlungen * Mach, Ernst Die Principien der Wärmelehre * Mausbach, Joseph Die Ethik des heiligen Augustinus. Erster Band: Die sittliche Ordnung und ihre Grundlagen * Mauthner, Fritz Die drei Bilder der Welt - ein sprachkritischer Versuch * Meissner, Franz Hermann Arnold Böcklin * Meyer, Elard Hugo Indogermanische Mythen, Bd. 1: Gandharven-Kentauren * Müller, Adam Versuche einer neuen Theorie des Geldes * Müller, Conrad Alexander von Humboldt und das Preußische Königshaus. Briefe aus den Jahren 1835-1857 * Oettingen, Arthur von Die Schule der Physik * Ostwald, Wilhelm Erfinder und Entdecker * Peters, Carl Die deutsche Emin-Pascha-Expedition * Poetter, Friedrich Christoph Logik * Popken, Minna Im Kampf um die Welt des Lichts. Lebenserinnerungen und Bekenntnisse einer Ärztin * Prutz, Hans Neue Studien zur Geschichte der Jungfrau von Orléans * Rank, Otto Psychoanalytische Beiträge zur Mythenforschung. Gesammelte Studien aus den Jahren 1912 bis 1914. * Ree, Paul Johannes Peter Candid * Rohr, Moritz von Joseph Fraunhofers Leben, Leistungen und Wirksamkeit * Rubinstein, Susanna Ein individualistischer Pessimist: Beitrag zur Würdigung Philipp Mainländers * Eine Trias von Willensmetaphysikern: Populär-philosophische Essays * Sachs, Eva Die fünf platonischen Körper: Zur Geschichte der Mathematik und der Elementenlehre Platons und der Pythagoreer * Scheidemann, Philipp Memoiren eines Sozialdemokraten, Erster Band * Memoiren eines Sozialdemokraten, Zweiter Band * Schleich, Carl Ludwig Erinnerungen an Strindberg nebst Nachrufen für Ehrlich und von Bergmann * Schlösser, Rudolf Rameaus Neffe - Studien und Untersuchungen zur Einführung in Goethes Übersetzung des Diderotschen Dialogs * Schweitzer, Christoph Reise nach Java und Ceylon (1675-1682). Reisebeschreibungen von deutschen Beamten und Kriegsleuten im Dienst der niederländischen West- und Ostindischen Kompagnien 1602 - 1797. * Sommerlad, Theo Die soziale Wirksamkeit der Hohenzollern * Stein, Heinrich von Giordano Bruno. Gedanken über seine Lehre und sein Leben * Strache, Hans Der Eklektizismus des Antiochus von Askalon * Sulger-Gebing, Emil Goethe und Dante * Thiersch, Hermann Ludwig I von Bayern und die Georgia Augusta * Pro Samothrake * Tyndall, John Die Wärme betrachtet als eine Art der Bewegung, Bd. 1 * Die Wärme betrachtet als eine Art der Bewegung, Bd. 2 * Virchow, Rudolf Vier Reden über Leben und Kranksein * Vollmann, Franz Über das Verhältnis der späteren Stoa zur Sklaverei im römischen Reiche * Wachsmuth, Curt Das alte Griechenland im neuen * Weber, Paul Beiträge zu Dürers Weltanschauung * Wecklein, Nikolaus Textkritische Studien zu den griechischen Tragikern * Weinhold, Karl Die heidnische Totenbestattung in Deutschland * Wellhausen, Julius Israelitische und Jüdische Geschichte, Reihe ReligioSus Band VI *Wellmann, Max Die pneumatische Schule bis auf Archigenes - in ihrer Entwickelung dargestellt * Wernher, Adolf Die Bestattung der Toten in Bezug auf Hygiene, geschichtliche Entwicklung und gesetzliche Bestimmungen * Weygandt, Wilhelm Abnorme Charaktere in der dramatischen Literatur. Shakespeare - Goethe - Ibsen - Gerhart Hauptmann * Wlassak, Moriz Zum römischen Provinzialprozeß * Wulffen, Erich Kriminalpädagogik: Ein Erziehungsbuch * Wundt, Wilhelm Reden und Aufsätze * Zallinger, Otto Die Ringgaben bei der Heirat und das Zusammengeben im mittelalterlich-deutschem Recht * Zoozmann, Richard Hans Sachs und die Reformation - In Gedichten und Prosastücken, Reihe ReligioSus Band III